DATE			

Drug Use in Pregnancy: Mother and Child

To Carol,
a very special person.

With love

Drug Use in Pregnancy: Mother and Child

Editor

Ira J. Chasnoff, MD
Assistant Professor of Pediatrics
and Psychiatry and Behavioral Sciences
Northwestern University Medical School
Chicago, Illinois

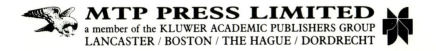

MTP PRESS LIMITED
a member of the KLUWER ACADEMIC PUBLISHERS GROUP
LANCASTER / BOSTON / THE HAGUE / DORDRECHT

Published in the UK and Europe by
MTP Press Limited
Falcon House
Lancaster, England

British Library Cataloguing in Publication Data

Drug use in pregnancy : mother and child.
1. Drug abuse in pregnancy
2. Fetus—Effects of drugs on 3. Infants
(Newborn)—Effects of drugs on
I. Chasnoff, Ira J.
618.3'2   RG580.D76

ISBN 0-85200-949-6

Published in the USA by
MTP Press
A division of Kluwer Academic Publishers
101 Philip Drive
Norwell, MA 02061, USA

Library of Congress Cataloging-in-Publication Data

Drug use in pregnancy.

Includes bibliographies and index.
1. Drug abuse in pregnancy.   2. Fetus—Effect of
drugs on.   3. Maternal–fetal exchange.
4. Infants (Newborn)—Effects of drugs on.
5. Pregnant women—Drug use.
I. Chasnoff, Ira J. [DNLM: 1. Fetus—drug
effects.   2. Infant, Newborn—drug effects.
3. Maternal–Fetal Exchange—drug effects.
4. Substance Abuse—in pregnancy.
5. Substance Dependence—in pregnancy.
WQ 200 D7943]
RG580.D76D79   1986   618.3'2   86-10395

ISBN 0-85200-949-6

Photoset by Chippendale Type,
Otley, West Yorkshire.
Printed by Anchor Brendon, Tiptree, Essex.

Contents

Foreword

With the emergence of the biological sciences in the seventeenth and eighteenth centuries, some explanations of congenital malformations with a basis in scientific fact were formulated. It was not, however, until the thalidomide tragedy in 1961 that the necessity for further study of the effects of environmental factors on congenital malformations was recognized. By the early 1970s concentrated efforts had begun to be directed toward evaluating the effects on the unborn child of mood-altering drugs taken during pregnancy. Over the past decade, research and treatment programs have led to the recognition of a full range of psychoactive drugs that affect the developing fetus either somatically or behaviorally. Programs for the treatment of the pregnant drug addict have been developed which concentrate not only on the pharmacologic therapy of the woman but also on the social and psychologic characteristics that place her and her unborn child at risk. This book is an attempt to bring together clinicians and researchers who have been active in developing programs for the recognition and management of the chemically dependent pregnant woman and her newborn. The contributions of the multiple disciplines which the authors represent emphasize the need for a multifactorial approach to the problems of drug use and abuse during pregnancy. It is hoped that through this type of approach a better future for substance-exposed infants, innocent bystanders in the process of addiction, can be assured.

Ira J. Chasnoff

Contributing Authors

I. J. CHASNOFF, MD
Perinatal Services
Chemical Dependence Program
Northwestern Memorial Hospital
320 East Huron Street
Chicago, IL 60611
USA

J. A. BIANCHI, RN
Perinatal Services
Chemical Dependence Program
Northwestern Memorial Hospital
320 East Huron Street
Chicago, IL 60611
USA

K. A. BURNS, PhD
Prentice Women's Hospital
330 East Superior Street
Chicago, IL 60611
USA

W. J. BURNS, PhD
Prentice Women's Hospital
330 East Superior Street
Chicago, IL 60611
USA

G. M. CHISUM, RN
Chemical Dependence Program
Northwestern Memorial Hospital
320 East Huron Street
Chicago, IL 60611
USA

G. P. DAVIS, MD
Institute of Psychiatry
Northwestern Memorial Hospital
320 East Huron Street
Chicago, IL 60611
USA

W. DONALD, MD
Prentice Women's Hospital
320 East Superior Street
Chicago, IL 60611
USA

P. A. FRIED, PhD
Department of Psychology
Carleton University
Ottawa, Ontario
K1S 5B6
Canada

R. S. IENNARELLA, PhD
Chemical Dependence Program
Northwestern Memorial Hospital
320 East Huron Street
Chicago, IL 60611
USA

K. KAYE, PhD
Department of Psychiatry
Northwestern University Medical School
320 East Huron Street
Chicago, IL 60611
USA

L. KEITH, MD
Prentice Women's Hospital
330 East Superior Street
Chicago, IL 60611
USA

L. L. KERNS, MD
Institute of Psychiatry
Northwestern Memorial Hospital
320 East Huron Street
Chicago, IL 60611
USA

A. O. MARTIN, PhD
Prentice Women's Hospital
330 East Superior Street
Chicago, IL 60611
USA

M. MITCHELL, MD
Prentice Women's Hospital
330 East Superior Street
Chicago, IL 60611
USA

K. C. RICH, MD
Department of Pediatrics
University of Illinois at Chicago
840 South Wood Street
Chicago, IL 60612
USA

M. ROSNER, MD
Prentice Women's Hospital
330 East Superior Street
Chicago, IL 60611
USA

S. H. SCHNOLL, MD
Department of Psychiatry
Northwestern Memorial Hospital
Superior Street and Fairbanks Court
Chicago, IL 60611
USA

M. J. WIET, JD
Northwestern Memorial Hospital
Superior Street and Fairbanks Court
Chicago, IL 60611
USA

Introduction:
The Genesis of Mother – Infant Interaction: How Parents Create Persons

KENNETH KAYE

In the past 10–15 years drug use in our society has increased among women of childbearing age. Concurrently our understanding of the dangers posed by any extreme disruption of fetal life, childbirth, or postnatal care has deepened by an order of magnitude. We have a more comprehensive view of the effects babies, and mothers and fathers, normally have upon one another. Therefore the task of pediatricians, nurses, and psychologists concerned with helping addicted neonatal families is more complex than it was thought to be 15 years ago. The intricacies of the social interactions through which the human mind is acquired, the turn-taking structure which characterizes these interactions from the beginning, the fact that all human parents constantly provide a framework of experiences for their infants' encounters with the physical as well as the social world, and the sensitive use that a normal mother or father makes of those innate properties of infant behavior to gradually construct meaningful communicative exchanges long before the baby even understands what meaning is: all these aspects of human development are relevant to concerns regarding the effects of maternal substance abuse on the developing fetus and child.

THE PARENT – INFANT SYSTEM

Normal human development begins within the context of a system of parental and/or family interaction. What has been learned from observations of parent–infant play is that parents instinctively do many things which help an infant emit behaviors that are actually beyond the capability of the infant alone. Infant development continues to unfold and progress within a context in which the infant is an apprentice to the parents. In this way a parent is like a master shoemaker who begins his teaching by setting up small tasks which are slightly beyond his apprentice's competence. The shoemaker closely supervises the apprentice's work and intervenes when necessary, or gives additional details when the apprentice appears ready. Often this help is offered in anticipation of problems in order to assure positive experiences for the apprentice, thereby reinforcing the apprentice's confidence to expand his own competence further. It is within this apprenticeship setting that parents and other caretakers provide for infants. It is this structuring framework that is species-specific and instinctive for humans and, therefore, universally present in human parenting. Such parenting behaviors constitute the environment of every human infant, whether extremely advantaged or disadvantaged. However, these behaviors may be presented with greater or less sensitivity to the child's needs at the moment, with greater or less consistency, and with accurate or inaccurate readings of a baby's intentions and skill. Thus, these behaviors are processes susceptible to impairment.

The most common setting in which mother–infant interaction has been studied has been during face-to-face play. Results of these studies have identified predictable patterns of interaction within normal mother–infant dyads. At 2 months of age it is the mother who initiates greetings when eye contact is made. As the infant matures such greetings begin to be initiated by the baby. Researchers call this communicative setting the 'dialogue frame'; it is a focus of mother and infant on one another with readiness to communicate. The dialogue frame begins with a mother talking to an infant *in utero* and continues with turn-taking during the pseudo-dialogues in face-to-face play. This dialogue frame will turn into real dialogue as soon as the infant is old enough to talk, but in the meantime it evolves into other kinds of frames which, we believe, are crucial to the infant's cognitive development.

An example of a commonly observed pattern of interactional behavior in normal mother–infant dyads is the 'instrumental frame.' An illustration of this pattern would be the case of an infant placing shapes into matching holes in a sphere. In early infancy a baby is only able to be successful at such a task if his mother rotates the sphere to present the correctly shaped hole in front of him. This 'instrumental frame' is also demonstrated in the behavior of a mother who steadies a tower of blocks each time her infant places a new one on the top. Caretakers very often provide this type of active guidance of an infant's behavior without any awareness that they are doing so. This guidance or 'instrumental frame' makes it possible for infants to be more effective at performing tasks than they would be by themselves.

It has often been observed that, even in the case of normal mother–infant interaction, difficulties may arise which interfere with the smooth ongoing dialogue. A normal infant is not always ready to respond to his mother's invitation to interact each time she gazes at the infant's face. It is understandable that this rejection of maternal gaze by the infant can be upsetting to some mothers, especially to those who are already anxious about mothering, or who themselves are going through personal distress or psychological maladjustment. An effective mother, however, tends to

2

accept the cycles of attention from her infant as normal variation, and to fit them into her maternal dialogue whenever the baby gives her an opportunity. Therefore it is normal for mothers to continue using the dialogue frame and the instrumental frame over many months of interaction until the infant learns to become more independent at emitting behaviors. For example, when the infant is 2 months of age a mother may pretend with her infant that they are holding hands and that they are talking to each other. Microanalysis of such sequences at that age shows that babies do not really initiate greetings but that mothers structure their own greetings in such a way that there is a high likelihood of eliciting a response from the infant. After 3 months of this maternal guidance, when this same infant has reached 5 months of age, it is then the infant who is initiating vocal greetings and smiling just as often as the mother.

APPRENTICESHIP

The theory that early human development proceeds as an apprenticeship is a way of integrating findings from studies of mother – infant interaction. The apprenticeship is made up of a series of stages. The first stage during the first 2 months of life is a period of 'shared rhythms and regulations' in which the intrinsic self-regulatory processes of the neonate are marshalled by extrinsic functions residing in the adult of the species. The second stage, from 2 to 8 months, is a period of 'shared intentions,' when adults infer what the baby is trying to accomplish and enable him to begin to fulfill intentions. He is thus able to practice the sensory-motor schemas which are constituent modules of more and more intelligent acts, as Piaget[1] and Bruner[2] have shown.

The period of 'shared memory' begins at about 8 months, when infants and parents begin playing stereotypic games remembered from one day to the next by both partners, yet still depending upon the parent's greater responsibility for simplifying, structuring, and suggesting. Finally, in the second year comes the period of 'shared language,' by which time the baby is not only comprehending and producing gestures within dyadic relationships but is a self-conscious member of the family system.

THE HIGH-RISK SYSTEM

The quality of parenting shown by human mothers varies widely, with comfortable, confident mothers at one end of the spectrum and anxious, depressed, neurotic mothers at the other end. In general, mothers differ most widely in the efficacy or effectiveness of their interactional behaviors and in the elegance or smoothness with which they orchestrate the synchrony of the relationship. Therefore any investigation of deviant mother–infant interaction must necessarily take into consideration the complexities of the interactional components involved in a mother–infant relationship. It would be convenient if one could simply predict that any baby whose physical system has been affected by his mother's chemical dependence will fail to elicit appropriate reactions from his parents or fail to respond to his parents' elicitations. However, such

3

failings may be only one aspect of many interwoven events which make up interactional deficiencies.

It would be a vast oversimplification to conceptualize the problem of substance abuse in terms of effects of drugs upon the developing fetus and child and consider nothing more than that. This oversimplification fits the medical or linear cause/effect model. Admittedly, such a model provides a rationale for preventive medicine: keep pregnant women off drugs. It also provides a basis for intervention, but only for the baby. It suggests that our response should be to find the best possible medical treatment for the newborn, as well as psychological interventions to counteract any deficits in the development of the child's intellectual capacities or personality.

Whatever effects drug abuse has upon the fetus, its effects are likely to make themselves felt upon the developing child through a multi-layered interaction. The factors in that interaction include at least the following: the infant's neurological system, the parents' sensitivities, the infant's intelligence (i.e. his brain's ability to make sense of the cues his parents offer him), and the parents' expectations. All four of these factors must be kept in mind when evaluating chemically dependent newborns.

In regard to the first factor, neurologic status, the passively addicted newborn may not present to the mother as alertly or engagingly as a normal infant. One of the frequent findings of research with the 'high–risk infants' is that some of them are not fully 'there' for their parents to respond to. This problem has been at the center of Brazelton's[3] work at Harvard University for nearly 20 years: to know enough about the evaluation of newborns to be able to accurately predict their developmental course over the early weeks of life and thus be able to counsel parents regarding the strengths and weaknesses of their infant.

The second aspect of 'high-risk infants' is that the baby, and often the mother, requires extra hospital care. This interferes with the normal process of acquaintance for the two members of the dyad by keeping them apart and by labeling the baby as 'abnormal.' Thus, high-risk neonatal care distances an already at-risk mother from her infant.

The remaining factors, the baby's intelligence and the parents' expectations, add a further level of complexity to the notion of risk. The newborn's developmental tasks can be conceptualized in terms of entering the family system as a very deficient but stimulating organism, being co-opted by parental frames and only slowly becoming a full member of the system, a person with a mind and a sense of self[4]. This whole process of assimilation into the family system for the purpose of development has been provided for by human evolution, both in the form of neurological mechanisms present in the neonatal organism, which stimulate adults to act in the way the organism needs them to act, and also in the form of instincts in parents to provide the kinds of frames babies need in order to become persons.

Although parental behaviors are somewhat guided by instincts, as they are in the rest of the animal kingdom, human parental behaviors are often strongly influenced by socially acquired characteristics such as maternal

4

expectations for the baby. It may be these expectations on the part of drug-abusing mothers that guide many of their early interactive behaviors. Therefore, a baby born to a chemically dependent mother might be at risk for starting the interactive process with the handicap of negative maternal expectations, even if the baby has no physical or psychological effects of *in utero* drug exposure. Mothers who abuse drugs during pregnancy are often told that their baby will be at risk; these mothers assume that such a risk exists because they have seen warnings in the media about using drugs during pregnancy. Such an expectation, even in the absence of all other factors, would place the mother – infant relationship at high risk for dysfunction.

In reality, of course, drug-using mothers not only have these negative expectations, but their infants often confirm their worst fears, because they are sleepy, jittery, withdrawing and irritable. Repeated instances of under- and over-responsiveness from her infant may prematurely convince even a patient mother that her infant is impaired, retarded or in pain, and that it is her fault. Worse yet, some mothers may begin to believe that the infant is showing intentional rejection.

This downward spiral of negative effects can be intensified if the mother herself is deficient in self-esteem. Such a case would be missed in the linear or medical model. Overly simplistic cause/effect thinking omits the factors leading to or complicating the mother's drug dependence: her addictive personality, poverty, emotional deprivation, ignorance and a whole host of indicators of poor readiness to be a parent. Whichever of these factors operates in a particular pregnant woman, and in her spouse or nuclear family, will be vital aspects of the social system into which the baby is born, even if that baby is medically protected from the mother's substance abuse; indeed, even if the mother's chemical dependence is treated before she conceives.

THE PROBLEM OF DRUG ABUSE

It appears that the frequency and severity of the problem of drug abuse in pregnancy continue to grow. Researchers are faced with a number of critical issues in relation to this problem. Which developmental processes in the exposed infant are affected most? Are there critical periods for the fetus or the embryo? What are the subtle effects which combine with maternal characteristics to affect such complex processes as mother–infant interaction? It is the hope that in the following pages we will ask these questions in such a way as to stimulate more productive investigations and more precise formulations of the questions themselves. Protecting an infant from the effects of illicit substance use by its mother protects it from being affected by only one aspect of a multidetermined pathological system. It is the pathological system, not the drug use alone, which must be addressed in any therapeutic endeavor.

REFERENCES

1. Piaget, J. (1952). *The Origins of Intelligence in Children.* (New York: International Universities Press)
2. Bruner, J. (1972). The nature and uses of immaturity. *American Psychologist,* **27,** 688 – 704
3. Brazelton, T. B. (1976). *Neonatal Behavioral Assessment Scale.* (Philadelphia: Spastics International Medical Publications)
4. Kaye, K. (1982). *The Mental and Social Life of Babies: How Parents Create Persons.* (Chicago: University of Chicago Press)

1
Pharmacologic Basis of Perinatal Addiction

SIDNEY H. SCHNOLL

The use and abuse of drugs during pregnancy occur more frequently than is generally realized. In studies attempting to look at the incidence of drug use during pregnancy, it has been reported that as many as 60% of pregnant women use some medications during their pregnancy[1-8]. The drugs used are primarily over-the-counter analgesics, antinauseants and sleep medications. The research investigating the use of drugs during pregnancy is often retrospective, based on the recall of the pregnant woman during or after pregnancy. Despite the information indicating high levels of drug use during pregnancy, few studies have systematically looked at urine toxicology during prenatal visits to verify the type and extent of drug use[9].

PERINATAL PHARMACOLOGY

To understand the effects of drug use during pregnancy, it is necessary to look at the maternal–placental–fetal unit. This unit consists of the mother, the placenta and the fetus, with each exerting some actions on drugs and influencing the total effect. Since the mother can be studied directly through easily obtained blood samples, it is easiest to study the pharmacokinetics and pharmacology of drugs in the mother and more difficult to study the placenta and the fetus.

Because of the numerous problems involved in collecting data on drug use during pregnancy, and the inability to perform the types of research on the fetus that would give us more information about effects on embryonic and fetal development, little human data is available. Animal studies are difficult to extrapolate to humans since there is extensive evidence indicating that the effects of drugs on fetal development in animals may not relate to the effects of the same drugs in humans[10].

The time during pregnancy that a drug is taken is extremely critical[11]. The first 8 weeks of pregnancy, before the woman knows she is pregnant, are usually the most critical in terms of embryonic development. Drugs

7

that severely affect the embryonic development at this point in the pregnancy usually cause a spontaneous abortion. The woman may not even know that she was pregnant except that she has missed one or more menstrual periods. Even though an early abortion may be the result of drug use, it is rarely considered as drug-induced. This limits our understanding of the effects of drugs on the early stages of pregnancy. To understand the pharmacologic actions of drugs it is important to understand drug pharmacokinetics. Several excellent reviews describe the complex interactions affecting the disposition of drugs in the maternal – placental – fetal unit during pregnancy[12–14].

Maternal factors

The route of administration of a drug influences its ability to cross the placenta. Drugs taken orally may undergo a significant first-pass metabolism in the liver. The drug may be metabolized to an ionized form, enhancing urinary excretion and reducing its ability to cross the placenta. If the drug is metabolized to a nonionized form its ability to cross the placenta will be increased. Drugs taken intramuscularly, intravenously or by inhalation do not undergo first-pass metabolism and may more readily cross the placenta following absorption from the site of administration.

Pregnancy can alter the woman's response with certain drugs. During pregnancy there is often decreased gastrointestinal motility, alterations in gastric pH and buffer capacity and increased mucous secretions. These effects will result in changes in absorption for many drugs. Alterations in venous pressure late in pregnancy can reduce the absorption of intramuscularly administered drugs. Plasma proteins gradually decrease during pregnancy; this decreases protein binding, making more free drug available[15]. In addition, increases in total body water and fat also alter drug disposition. As pregnancy advances there is an increase in glomerular filtration resulting in increased drug excretion.

Increased progesterone levels during pregnancy cause an induction of liver enzymes, often resulting in increased hepatic metabolism of drugs.

Some of these changes can increase the amount of drug reaching the fetus, and others can decrease it. The changes occurring in a specific woman can be quite variable, and the effects of these changes on a given drug would relate to the nature of that specific drug. It is therefore difficult to predict from the changes described exactly which effects will occur.

Placental factors

There is a misconception that the placenta blocks drugs from crossing from the maternal to the fetal circulation, therefore protecting the fetus from their noxious effects[16]. All drugs are able to cross the placenta to some extent, especially if given in large quantities over a prolonged period of time. There are several factors known to enhance the ability of a drug to cross the placenta, lipid solubility and a molecular weight of less than 1000 being the most important. These two factors also increase the ability of a drug to cross the blood–brain barrier into the central nervous system. A simple rule of thumb is that any drug that crosses the blood–brain barrier and has an effect on the central nervous system of the mother will also cross the placenta.

Most drugs are distributed throughout the body bound to plasma proteins. The ratio of free to bound drug influences the quantity of drug crossing the placenta. Drugs bound to serum proteins are unable to cross the placenta because of the size of the drug–protein complex. Only unbound, free drug can cross the placenta. Displacing a drug from its protein binding site increases the amount of free drug, and therefore increases the amount of drug able to cross the placenta. The serum pH also may affect the state in which the drug exists. If a drug is in an ionized state it will not easily cross the placenta and is more likely to be highly protein-bound. Drugs in a nonionized state more readily cross the placenta[16].

The placenta is not a passive, sieve-like structure but an active organ which has many metabolic functions. Recent studies have indicated that the placenta is able to produce enzymes involved in oxidation, reduction, hydrolysis and conjugation of drugs[17].

Fetal factors

Little is known about the functions of the human fetus in relation to drugs. However, recent studies indicate that the fetus is capable of some metabolic activity at relatively early stages of gestation[17]. These studies indicate that the fetus and placenta can metabolize drugs but there are low levels of glucuronyl transferases, resulting in a failure to terminate the biological effects of drugs. Further investigation of these findings is necessary to determine their significance.

TERATOLOGY

The major concern of drug use during pregnancy is the effects that the drugs might have on fetal development. Although the rate of congenital malformations noted at the time of birth is relatively low, about 2–3%, this figure may be inaccurate because some malformations do not appear until later in life[18]. An example of this is the effect of diethylstilbestrol taken during pregnancy on later carcinoma of the uterus[19]. Because these effects occur long after the drug was taken, they might not be associated with drug use during pregnancy, and therefore are not classified as teratologic effects of the drug.

The most obvious problems associated with drugs taken during pregnancy are dysmorphic effects. The development of teratologic changes is dependent on a number of variables[11]. Most significantly, for any given drug there is a threshold level at which the malformations may occur. In order to achieve this threshold level the drug has to be taken in a sufficient dose and over a sufficient duration for that level to accumulate in the fetus. In addition, the fetus must be genetically susceptible to the effects of the drug. The importance of genetic susceptibility is becoming clearer as we study large populations using various drugs during

9

pregnancy. Not all of the embryos and fetuses exposed to the drug develop the problems. Therefore, there has to be some level of fetal susceptibility.

The drug itself plays an important role in the development of teratologic effects, particularly the pharmacologic and physicochemical properties of the drug and its metabolites. The drug has to interact with the developing embryo and fetus in a way that arrests or alters certain developmental patterns, resulting in the teratologic effect[11].

Maternal factors may also play a role in the development of dysmorphic teratology[11]. Increasing maternal age increases the possibility of teratologic effects. Diet can be very important; improper nutrition can result in developmental abnormalities. The condition of the uterus also plays a role. If there are malformations in the uterus or problems with uterine function, teratologic effects can occur. Hormonal balance and diseases in the mother may also affect fetal development. Rubella and other diseases have been identified as causing developmental abnormalities. External factors have also been shown to be important in fetal development. Socioeconomics, climate, altitude and other factors can play a role that affects the developing fetus. All of these factors can coalesce in an interactive way resulting in fetal abnormalities. The timing of a particular event during pregnancy is critical in relation to teratology. A drug administered early during embryonic development can cause marked teratologic effects, whereas the same drug administered later in fetal development may have no effect whatsoever.

Dysmorphic teratology is considered to be the major problem associated with drug use during pregnancy, but recently there has been increased concern over behavioral teratology. This is usually less obvious and, therefore, is not as easily recognized as dysmorphic teratology. Behavioral teratology is less well understood, and in recent years the development of neonatal behavioral assessment scales and other tests looking at behavior of the newborn have helped us to delineate behavioral teratology[20].

The factors causing behavioral teratology are the same as those discussed above for dysmorphic teratology. In addition to the effects on development, direct effects of the drug due to persistence in the newborn or the presence of withdrawal effects due to fetal dependence can alter the behavioral tests. The fetus accumulates certain drugs because of their pharmacokinetic characteristics; therefore the drugs may still be exerting an effect on the newborn. Thus, any measurements of behavior may not truly be measuring teratologic effects but may be measuring the effect of the drug on the fetus at that time.

In addition to drug effects interfering with the determination of behavioral teratology, parenting problems can also be involved. Once the newborn is delivered, the interactions with the parent can markedly alter newborn and infant development, and tests for alterations in behavior may not be truly measuring teratologic effects but could be measuring parental influence on behavior.

Drugs teratogenic to the fetus usually have no harmful effects on the mother. Often, these drugs are beneficial to the mother and may be necessary to alleviate maternal medical problems. Therefore it becomes a delicate balance when prescribing a drug to counteract certain problems in the mother that may have severe consequences on fetal development.

Teratologic effects seem to be more prevalent if drugs are taken during the embryonic stage of development[11]. This is during the first 8 – 12 weeks of development, when the mother may not be aware that she is pregnant. Because of the enormous amount of tissue differentiation taking place during this period, and the organic development occurring, the embryo is very susceptible to drugs. The embryo at this stage of development has incomplete metabolic and excretory functions so drugs tend to accumulate rather than being removed[17].

During the fetal stage the most common drug effect is growth retardation[11]. Again, limited fetal metabolic and excretory functions have developed at this point. With the considerable brain development taking place during this period it is also possible that, in addition to dysmorphic teratology, this is the stage of development when behavioral teratologic effects occur[21]. Behavioral effects can also occur during the neonatal stage, because of immature function of organs, delaying excretion of various drugs[22]. Studies have shown that diazepam administered during labor in a single dose takes from 10 to 18 days to be excreted by the neonate[23]. Meperidine is excreted over a 5–7-day period[24], and recent studies have shown that cocaine takes 3–5 days to be excreted by the neonate[25]. These slow excretion times for drugs can result in prolonged drug effects, interference with behavioral assessment scales, and withdrawal syndromes occurring weeks to months after delivery. These withdrawal syndromes may affect brain development occurring post-delivery.

DRUGS OF ABUSE

Most research studying drug use during pregnancy has been an attempt to monitor prescription or over-the-counter drugs taken by the mother, or studies of animals given specific drugs. However, an abuser of illicit drugs during pregnancy places another burden on the ability to study the effects of these drugs on embryonic, fetal and neonatal development. Street drug use often means that the person has no idea of the drug being taken[26]. Studies over the past few years have demonstrated that, in many cases, drugs purchased on the street do not contain the substances that are believed to be in them. Caffeine, pseudoephedrine and phenylpropanolamine are often sold as amphetamine. Valium is often sold as Quaalude, and street THC is almost always phencyclidine (PCP)[27,28]. Because of this widespread substitution it is difficult to determine from history exactly what the patient has taken and, therefore, information provided by the patient should be verified by urine toxicology.

Probably the greatest problem associated with street drugs is the presence of contaminants. With the variable purity of street drugs, they are often cut with other substances. These substances can be other drugs or relatively inert substances such as sugars or talcum powder. When other drugs are present the contaminating drugs could be a more serious threat to health than the drug the person thought s/he was buying[26]. A common contaminant of many street drugs is phencyclidine because of its low cost and widespread availability[28]. In almost all cases the street drugs contain materials other than the substances they are supposed to contain. These materials may be teratogenic in their own right or result in interactions having teratogenic potential.

With the problems discussed above for street drugs it is often very difficult to determine exactly what substance may have caused a teratologic problem. Therefore large numbers of patients must be studied, and it is necessary to do frequent analyses of urine and blood to determine exactly what drugs were being taken and, if possible, samples of street drugs should be obtained to determine what is being sold on the street.

Urine toxicology can be of great importance in determining precisely what drug was taken. However, it is not helpful in determining how much or how often the drug was taken. A positive urine toxicology reveals only that a given drug was taken within the time period that the drug can be detected in the urine. Various methods are currently being used to screen urines, and each of these methods has pros and cons. Two of the most important factors involved in evaluating toxicologic procedures are sensitivity and specificity.

Sensitivity refers to how sensitive the technique is in recognizing the presence of a given drug or metabolite. Screening procedures should be very sensitive so that no positives are missed. The problem with very sensitive screening techniques is the high frequency of false-positive results. Because of the false-positives, all positives from a sensitive screening procedure should be verified on a second testing procedure that is less sensitive but more specific for the substance producing the positive result on the screening procedure. Highly sensitive screening tests for drugs in urine include thin-layer chromatography and immunoassay techniques.

Specificity refers to how specific a test is in determining the presence of a given drug to the exclusion of other drugs. A highly specific test should have few false-positive results. The tests with high specificity are often poor screening tests because they usually can identify only one substance at a time and are often more expensive than the screening tests. These tests are used to confirm positive results from screening procedures. If the result is not positive on both tests it should be considered a negative finding. Currently, gas-chromatography/mass-spectrometry, high-performance liquid chromatography and gas-chromatography are used in confirmatory testing. Immunoassays can also be used in some cases.

TREATMENT

Because of the enormous problems associated with the use of street drugs, one of the approaches to treatment of the chemically dependent pregnant woman is to place her on an alternative drug that will hopefully reduce street drug use. The most commonly used drug at the present time is methadone, which is utilized in the treatment of opiate-dependent women[29]. Methadone is useful because it is long-acting, and therefore a woman is able to maintain fairly consistent blood levels in contrast to utilizing opiates on the street which are usually short-acting, resulting in wide swings in blood levels. These rapid swings from intoxication to withdrawal can have severe adverse effects on the fetus, often producing premature labor and spontaneous abortions. Methadone also reduces street use of opiates and other drugs by blocking withdrawal and craving. Street heroin is frequently 'cut' with substances such as quinine or procaine, which can have teratogenic effects.

In opioid-dependent pregnant women, one of the major problems is determining the dose of methadone required to block withdrawal and craving without producing intoxication. Often the information available from the patient exaggerates the amount of drug she is taking on the street. Upon entering treatment, most drug abusers will report the greatest amount of drug ever used as the average amount used. A simple method of verifying daily usage is to take a detailed history of the amount used in the 24 hours prior to presenting for treatment. This figure is usually closer to the average daily use. By comparing the use in the previous 24 hours with the patient's current state of withdrawal or intoxication it is possible to estimate the patient's true use pattern. An example would be a patient who claims to use 20 bags of heroin a day, but in the previous 24 hours has only used 4 bags and has not used any heroin for 6 hours prior to her examination. Her examination reveals no signs of withdrawal. This would confirm that 4 bags is closer to her average daily dose. In addition, by knowing the current quality of street heroin (the average percentage of heroin in each bag), the dose of methadone can be determined.

With heroin samples running 2–3% purity, a dose of methadone of 2 mg/bag is usually sufficient to prevent withdrawal and reduce craving. The patient should then be monitored daily at the beginning of treatment for signs of intoxication or withdrawal, and dosage adjustments made accordingly. In cases where intoxication is present, the urine toxicology can be helpful in determining if the intoxication is due to methadone or other abused agents.

Once the patient is stabilized on a dose of methadone it is possible to gradually reduce the dose without creating problems for the mother or fetus. When reducing methadone levels in a pregnant woman, inform the patient that the dose will be changed but do not inform her of the amount it will be reduced or the rate of reduction. By keeping the patient blind to the dose, anxiety is reduced.

Decreasing the dose of methadone 1 mg a day in a blind fashion produces a smooth withdrawal without adverse fetal effects. Although not recommended, we have withdrawn women who have requested it at the above rate with no ill-effects. The rate of withdrawal should be altered if the patient shows signs of abstinence or there is an indication of fetal distress.

13

Some investigators have reported the need to increase the dose of methadone in the third trimester to maintain the pregnant addict without signs of withdrawal[30]. This is not consistent with experience of our program. We find that a reduction in methadone during the third trimester reduces the incidence of neonatal withdrawal.

Experience has demonstrated that a methadone dose of less than 20 mg per day at the time of delivery significantly reduces the presence of neonatal withdrawal signs and symptoms. Every effort should therefore be made to place the patient on the lowest possible dose of methadone to reduce continued street drug use and eliminate signs of withdrawal. Although the immediate withdrawal reaction is significantly reduced in the neonate with lower doses of methadone, there is a persistent protracted abstinence syndrome lasting from 4 to 6 months, demonstrated by the persistence of the Moro reaction in infants born to mothers who have been taking methadone[31].

Despite widespread use of alcohol, sedative-hypnotics and stimulants during pregnancy, there are no maintenance drugs currently accepted for the treatment of women dependent on these other substances. Phenobarbital and benzodiazepines have been used to withdraw women who have abused alcohol and sedative-hypnotics during pregnancy, but there are no studies documenting the effects of these drugs on withdrawal and long-term consequences. In patients abusing stimulant drugs the treatment of choice is a gradual reduction of the drug at a rate of from 5 to 10% per day of the total dose. This information is based on clinical experience in our own program and case reports. There are no studies that have carefully assessed withdrawal phenomena in women who are dependent on stimulant drugs.

With the evidence of behavioral effects of drug use during pregnancy, little is known about the underlying mechanisms of these behavioral changes. Currently, research is under way in our laboratory to investigate the effect of drug use during pregnancy on central nervous system neuroreceptors. Animal studies have demonstrated that pregnant dams placed on methadone produce pups that at 1 year of age show alterations in mu and delta opiate receptors in the hypothalamic region and no change in alpha-2 adrenergic receptors. In the cerebral cortex, pups that were prenatally exposed to methadone showed decreased delta and mu receptors and also decreased alpha-2 receptors. Postnatal exposure to methadone via breast feeding from a dam who is taking methadone results in decreased alpha-2 receptors in the cerebral cortex. These data demonstrate that in rats there are persistent central nervous system effects from *in utero* drug exposure. There is currently no evidence that similar effects occur in humans.

Much more research is necessary to determine if these alterations in receptors in the brain correlate with behavioral changes. Receptors in the central nervous system develop over a period of time, and some receptor systems are still developing postnatally. The time of exposure could be very critical in determining whether or not there are any behavioral effects.

14

CONCLUSIONS

Although it is well known that the effects on the fetus of drugs taken during pregnancy can be devastating, the amount of research that is currently available in humans is sparse, making it difficult to draw significant conclusions. Animal studies do not always correlate with human findings, making it difficult to interpret animal studies. Much more research is necessary to fully understand the consequences of drug use during pregnancy and how to effectively prescribe medication to pregnant women in order to reduce both dysmorphic and behavioral teratology.

REFERENCES

1. Fofar, J. O. and Nelson, M. M. (1973). Epidemiology of drugs taken by pregnant women: Drugs that may affect the fetus adversely. *Clin. Pharmacol. Ther.*, **14**, 632 – 42
2. Heinonen, O. P., Slone, D. and Shapiro, S. (1977). *Birth Defects and Drugs in Pregnancy*. (Littleton, MA: Publishing Sciences Group)
3. Brocklebank, J. C., Roy, W. A., Federspiel, C. I. and Schaffner, W. (1978). Drug prescribing during pregnancy: a controlled study of Tennessee Medicaid recipients. *Am. J. Obstet. Gynecol.*, **132**, 235 – 44
4. Kullander, R. and Kallen, B. (1976). A prospective study of drugs and pregnancy, Parts 1 – 4. *Acta Obstet. Gynecol. Scand.*, **55**, 25 – 33
5. Nora, J. J., Nora, A. H., Sommerville, R. J., Hill, R. M. and McNamara, D. G. (1967). Maternal exposure to potential teratogens. *J. Am. Med. Assoc.*, **202**, 1065 – 9
6. Rayburn, W., Wible-Kant, J. and Bledsoe, P. (1982). Changing trends in drug use during pregnancy. *J. Reprod. Med.*, **27**, 569 – 75
7. Jick, H., Holmes, L. B., Hunter, J. R., Madsen, S. and Stergackis, A. (1981). First-trimester drug use and congenital disorders. *J. Am. Med. Assoc.*, **246**, 343 – 6
8. Doering, P. L. and Stewart, R. B. (1978). The extent and character of drug consumption during pregnancy. *J. Am. Med. Assoc.*, **239**, 843 – 6
9. Hill, R. M. (1973). Drugs ingested by pregnant women. *Clin. Pharmacol. Ther.*, **14**, 454 – 9
10. Rudolph, A. M. (1985). Animal models for study of fetal drug exposure. In Chiang, C. N. and Lee, C. C. (eds) *Prenatal Drug Exposure: Kinetics and Dynamics, NIDA Research Monograph Series #60*, pp. 5 – 16. (Rockville, MD: US Department of Health and Human Services)
11. Tuchman-Duplessis, H. (1980). Embryonic clinical pharmacology. In Avery, G. S. (ed.) *Drug Treatment: Principles and Practice of Clinical Pharmacology and Therapeutics*, 2nd edn., pp. 62 – 75. (New York: ADIS Press)
12. Mirkin, B. L. (1976). *Perinatal Pharmacology and Therapeutics*. (New York: Academic Press)
13. Wang, L. H., Rudolph, A. M. and Benet, L. Z. (1980). Pharmacokinetics of drugs and metabolites in the maternal – placental – fetal unit: general principles. In Chiang, C. N. and Lee, C. C. (eds) *Prenatal Drug Exposure: Kinetics and Dynamics, NIDA Research Monograph Series #60*, pp. 25–38. (Rockville: MD, US Department of Health and Human Services)
14. Stock, B. H. (1981). Drug disposition in pregnancy. *Pharmacy Int.*, 60 – 3
15. Rebond, P., Groulade, J. and Groslambert, P. (1963). The influence of normal pregnancy and the post partum state on plasma proteins and lipids. *Am. J. Obstet. Gynecol.*, **86**, 820 – 32
16. Mirkin, B. L. and Singh, S. (1976). Placental transfer of pharmacologically active molecules. In Mirkin, B. L. (ed.) *Perinatal Pharmacology and Therapeutics*, pp. 1 – 69. (New York: Academic Press)
17. Juchau, M. R. (1985). Biotransformation of drugs and foreign chemicals in the human fetal-placental unit. In Chiang, C. N. and Lee, C. C. (eds.) *Prenatal Drug Exposure: Kinetics and Dynamics, NIDA Research Monograph Series #60*, pp. 17–24. (Rockville, MD: US Department of Health and Human Services)

18. Ash, P., Vennart, J. and Carter, O. D. (1977). The incidence of hereditary disease in man. *Lancet*, **1**, 849 – 51
19. Herbst, A. L., Cole, P., Colton, T., Robboy, S. J. and Scully, R. C. (1977). Age-incidence and risk of DES-related clear cell adenocarcinoma of the vagina and cervix. *Am. J. Obstet. Gynecol.*, **128**, 43 – 9
20. Brazelton, T. B. (1976). *Neonatal Behavioral Assessment Scale*, pp. 63–4. (Philadelphia: Spastics International Medical Publications)
21. Gal, P. and Sharpless, M. K. (1984). Fetal drug exposure—behavioral teratogenesis. *Drug Intell. Clin. Pharmacy*, **18**, 186 – 201
22. Morselli, P. L. (1976). Clinical pharmacokinetics in neonates. *Clin. Pharmacokinetics*, **1**, 81
23. Erkkola, R., Kanto, J. and Sellman, R. (1974). Diazepam in early human pregnancy. *Acta Obstet. Gynecol. Scand.*, **53**, 135 – 8
24. Caldwell, J., Wakile, L. A., Nortarianni, L. J., Smith, R. L., Correy, G. J., Lieberman, B. A., Beard, R. W., Finnie, M. D. A. and Snedden, W. (1978). Maternal and neonatal disposition of pethidine in childbirth: a study using quantitative gas chromatography/mass spectometry. *Life Sci.*, **22**, 589 – 96
25. Chasnoff, I. J., Bussey, M., Savich, R. and Stack, C. A. (1986). Perinatal cerebral infarction and maternal cocaine use. *J. Pediatr.* **108**, 456-9
26. Schnoll, S. H. (1979). Pharmacological aspects of youth drug abuse. In Beschner, G. M. and Friedman, A. S. (eds) *Youth Drug Abuse – Problems, Issues, and Treatment*, pp. 255 – 75. (Lexington, MA: Lexington Books)
27. Schnoll, S. H. and Vogel, W. H. (1974). Analysis of 'street drugs.' *N. Engl. J. Med.*, **284**, 781
28. Schnoll, S. H. (1980). Street PCP scene: issues on synthesis and contamination. *J. Psychedelic Drugs*, **12**, 229 – 33
29. Finnegan, L. P. (ed.) (1979). *Drug Dependency in Pregnancy: Clinical Management of Mother and Child. NIDA Services Research Monograph Series.* pp. 29 – 49. (Rockville, MD: US Department of Health, Education and Welfare)
30. Kreek, M. J. (1979). Methadone disposition during the perinatal period in humans. *Pharmacol. Biochem. Behav.*, **11**, 7 – 13
31. Chasnoff, I. J. and Burns, W. J. (1984). The Moro reaction: a scoring system for neonatal narcotic withdrawal. *Dev. Med. Child Neurol.*, **26**, 484 – 9

16

2
Recognition and Initial Management of the Pregnant Substance-abusing Woman

GAY M. CHISUM

Chemical dependence among women of childbearing age (18–34) continues to increase, and the substance abuse literature shows they are overrepresented among those persons who are current and regular users of legal drugs, illegal drugs and alcohol[1]. The pregnant substance-abusing patient is encountered in many settings including hospital medical units, obstetrical clinics, labor/delivery suites, postpartum units and in community liaison work. Due to the potential contact with this high-risk population, medical personnel should become aware of their attitudes toward this population, the skills and knowledge needed to identify these patients and the patients' referral needs. This paper will address the importance of early identification of the pregnant substance-abuser and will also briefly describe a model intervention procedure jointly used by the Prentice Women's Hospital and Maternity Center and Northwestern's Perinatal Services component of the Chemical Dependence Program of Northwestern University.

The pregnant substance-abusing patient may be easily overlooked, or, frequently, the patient may be identified but there is a lack of follow-through for referral to treatment. Many in the medical profession have had no orientation to perinatal addiction, which may account for lack of follow-through or inadequate chemical dependence assessments. Sokol *et al.*[2] suggest that 'clinicians are continuing to miss the diagnosis in at least three of every four alcohol-abusing patients. It is unlikely that there is any other OB/GYN diagnosis that is missed as often.' Although Sokol and Miller were concentrating on alcohol abuse, there are today few pure alcohol-abusing patients. Thus, chemical dependence can be seen as one of the most frequently missed diagnoses, specifically in pregnant women.

Medical personnel have an excellent opportunity to thoroughly evaluate the pregnant substance abuser. The clinical assessment for substance abuse should include an evaluation of the physical appearance, a medical and obstetrical history and a substance abuse interview.

PHYSICAL APPEARANCE

The evaluation of the patient's physical appearance begins with the initial introduction to the patient. The physical appearance may give subtle or overt clues to alert the interviewer to possible substance abuse. The following areas of concern should be noted:

1. Is the patient well-oriented?
2. Does the patient appear physically exhausted?
3. Are the patient's pupils extremely dilated or constricted?
4. Does the appearance of the patient's pregnancy coincide with the stated gestational age?
5. Are there signs of track marks, abscesses, edema in the upper or lower extremities?

The physical appearance and signs of chemical dependence are especially helpful in diagnosing the intravenous substance abuser. These women often seek acute medical treatment for complications of their chemical dependence due to their ambivalence toward the pregnancy coupled with their denial of chemical dependence; they frequently delay medical intervention until late in gestation. Medical staff find no history of prior obstetrical care. Some pregnant polydrug- and alcohol-abusing women may seek obstetrical care earlier in gestation. Since these women have less overt physical signs of chemical dependence, a very careful medical and obstetrical assessment is necessary.

MEDICAL HISTORY

In the medical history, an interviewer looks for the effects of substance abuse. A positive history for cirrhosis, hepatitis, bacterial endocarditis, cellulitis, pneumonia or pancreatitis should call attention to a possible history of substance abuse[3].

In a general medical unit, 25–40% of the admissions are due to the effects of chemical dependence[3,4]. Medical personnel must be willing to explore specific questions regarding prior hospitalization. A substance-abuser will volunteer little information; if past medical history appears negative, the pregnant woman's obstetrical history may be more revealing.

OBSTETRICAL HISTORY

As the interviewer proceeds to the obstetrical history, he/she should pay close attention to past and present information. Regardless of the patient's self-disclosure, the interviewer may discover prior complications due to perinatal substance abuse. These prior complications of pregnancy, labor or delivery require further exploration, and a request for past obstetrical records is indicated. Complications associated with drug use in pregnancy may include spontaneous abortion, premature labor, premature rupture of membranes, abruptio placentae, fetal death, meconium-stained amniotic fluid or a low birthweight infant[4].

Pertinent findings in regard to the present pregnancy may include poor weight gain, spotting or vaginal bleeding, an inactive fetus, reports of early contractions or a hyperactive fetus.

The obstetrical history also provides the interviewer with an opportunity to discuss the patient's emotional response to the current pregnancy. An inconsistent pattern of prenatal care may indicate apathy or ambivalence regarding the pregnancy. On the other hand, frequent emergency room visits may reveal extreme anxiety regarding the physical well-being of the fetus. In this setting the interviewer can explore the patient's coping mechanisms, exploring drug use during pregnancy and the potential risk to mother, fetus, newborn and the developing child. Past drug use is explored in a nonjudgmental manner while identifying early drug abuse patterns. The patient's substance abuse history should begin with the earliest exposure to cigarettes, over-the-counter medications, prescribed medications, alcohol, marijuana and other illicit drugs.

Substance abuse during past pregnancies

It is important to look at the substance abuse patterns during past pregnancies. Some women abstain from drugs during pregnancy while others curb drug use but return to drugs immediately postpartum. There are also women who have binges of substance abuse and others who are addicted to drugs regardless of their pregnancy. Some questions to be explored regarding past pregnancies are:

1. Did the patient experience any complications with the pregnancy, labor or delivery?
2. Did the patient's pediatrician notice any physical or behavioral problems with the newborn?
3. How is the child doing now? Does the patient notice any differences in behavior or growth patterns?

Current pregnancy

The current substance abuse history should begin at least 1 month prior to the last normal menstrual period. Many substance-abusing women do not have a regular menstrual cycle, and they often are unaware of a pregnancy until relatively late in gestation.

The current substance abuse history should include cigarettes, caffeine, all types of alcohol (beer, wine, mixed drinks, hard liquor and wine coolers), which may lead into the substance abuse interview.

SUBSTANCE ABUSE HISTORY

All prenatal history forms should include questions pertaining to chemicals used during pregnancy. Beginning a substance abuse history with cigarettes and proceeding to over-the-counter drugs, prescribed drugs, alcohol, marijuana and other illicit drugs appears less threatening to the patient. A positive substance abuse history requires immediate intervention by the medical staff.

INTERVENTION PROCEDURE

A medical intervention procedure can include patient confrontation, education, in-house or community referral to chemical dependence treatment, referral to a social worker or clinical nurse specialist for in-depth interviews and/or follow-up for treatment. Regardless of the type of intervention used, a patient should be strongly encouraged to follow through on treatment recommendations.

At Prentice Women's Hospital and Maternity Center, a past or present substance abuse history requires referral to Perinatal Services. The Perinatal Services Coordinator takes a more detailed chemical dependence history which includes past substance abuse, past pregnancies and substance abuse, and substance abuse during the current pregnancy. The Coordinator also focuses on the circumstances in which the drugs were taken and the problems encountered including physical, emotional, interpersonal, employment–vocational, family and legal.

Past substance abuse

The interviewer should begin with an explanation of the importance of prescribed drugs, illicit drugs and over-the-counter medications. It is important to obtain the most accurate daily, weekly and monthly substance abuse information.

Once the interviewer has collected the complete substance abuse history, explored the woman's current psychosocial stressors, investigated the circumstances surrounding her substance abuse and evaluated the effects of the substance abuse on the woman's life, treatment should be initiated.

Treatment

At Perinatal Services, treatment intervention begins with patient education regarding the possible effects on mother, fetus, newborn and developing child. The Coordinator initiates formal treatment for chemical dependence and makes a referral for routine obstetrical care at Prentice Women's Hospital.

Patient education

Most women are receptive to learning the possible effects of substance abuse on their pregnancy. Patient information is provided by use of diagrams, written materials and a discussion focusing on the patient's specific substance abuse patterns. Patient education may stimulate feelings of remorse; therefore the patient requires a great deal of emotional support from medical staff. It is important not only to help the women express their fears but also to refocus them on caring for the fetus from that point until delivery.

Formal treatment

The Perinatal Coordinator initiates treatment in inpatient or community chemical dependence programs when appropriate. At Northwestern Memorial Hospital the basic aspects of formal treatment in the Chemical Dependence Program include medical, psychotherapeutic and pharmacological services. Specific details of these services are outlined in other chapters. These services are provided in inpatient or outpatient programs with an interdisciplinary team approach to patient care. Northwestern University also has a specific Perinatal Services program for the chemically dependent pregnant woman. Perinatal Services, a comprehensive program, provides individual, group and family psychotherapy; prenatal education; prenatal care at Prentice Women's Hospital; Lamaze training; medication management; delivery at Prentice Women's Hospital; home nursing referral; infant developmental evaluation clinic; pediatric clinic; postpartum education classes; postpartum individual, group and family psychotherapy; and mother–infant interaction group.

There are women who choose not to accept chemical dependence treatment, although the Perinatal Coordinator strongly recommends treatment. Those women refusing treatment are referred to area hospitals which do not support a policy of identification and treatment for the pregnant substance abuser, although the women are given the same patient education and are also given the telephone number of Perinatal Services if they desire treatment in the future. If patients refuse treatment, documentation is necessary to alert others to the patients' status.

Referral to routine obstetrical care

Referrals are made back to Prentice Women's Hospital when a woman's history is negative for current chemical dependence, although some women may warrant follow-up with social work services due to a potential for returning to substance abuse under the stress of pregnancy. A nurse, social worker or physician can always refer a patient back to the Perinatal Coordinator for reevaluation.

It is important that medical personnel be familiar with perinatal addiction in order to meet the needs of the pregnant substance abuser. These patients require a genuine concern from medical staff, adequate time for thorough assessment, appropriate treatment referrals and active follow-up. The institutions initiating early identification procedures should see the outcome of decreased staff time and money in the care of pregnant chemically dependent women and their newborns in specialized units such as intensive care units or pediatric intensive care units.

REFERENCES

1. Chambers C. D. and Hart, L. G. (1977). Drug use patterns in pregnant women. In Rementeria, J. L. (ed.) *Drug Abuse in Pregnancy and Neonatal Effects,* pp. 73 – 81. (St Louis: Mosby)
2. Sokol, R. J., Miller, S. I. and Martier, S. (1981). *Preventing Fetal Alcohol Effects: a Practical Guide for OB/GYN Physicians and Nurses.* (Rockville, MD: National Institute on Alcohol Abuse and Alcoholism)
3. Finnegan, L. P. (ed.) (1979). *Drug Dependence in Pregnancy: Clinical Management of Mother and Child,* pp. 33 – 35. (Rockville, MD: National Institute on Drug Abuse)
4. Stark, M. J. and Nichols, H. G. (1977). Alcohol-related admissions to a general hospital. *Alc. Health Res. World,* (Summer), 11 – 14

3
Obstetric Aspects of Perinatal Addiction

LOUIS KEITH, WILLIE DONALD, MARVIN ROSNER,
MARILYN MITCHELL and JILL BIANCHI

INTRODUCTION

Despite the conspicuous absence of national and regional data on the numbers of addicted individuals (male or female), it is widely acknowledged that substance abuse has pervaded American society to an extent unparalleled in the history of this country. Reports of individuals addicted to traditional 'hard' as well as so-called 'recreational' drugs continually appear in the popular media. No socioeconomic level of society or racial or ethnic group has been spared, and the number of addicted pregnant women who have come to medical facilities for delivery in the past decade has risen substantially.

Prior to 1970 it was commonly believed that female opiate addicts were infertile. Two factors were thought to underlie this problem: (1) long-term abuse of opiates was associated with menstrual irregularities, oligo-ovulation and decreased libido[1]; and (2) since so many of these women of necessity resorted to prostitution to support their addictions, salpingitis and a variety of sexually transmitted infections were thought to add a tubal component to the presumed hormonal derangement. Since 1970, however, the concept that infertility was a foregone sequel of addiction in females has been reconsidered in light of studies which propose that methadone and heroin may actually be stimulators of ovulation[1]. In one report a three-fold increase in multiple births was actually observed[2]. Unfortunately, the problems inherent in following lifestyles are so complex as to make it unlikely in the foreseeable future that broad-based population studies will be able to generate definitive answers to questions regarding fertility rates for addicted women.

Whereas addiction to opiates and heroin was once the major clinical concern in programs devoted to the care of pregnant addicts[3], mixed (polydrug) substance abuse became relatively commonplace by 1975[4]. At

present, cocaine addiction (either alone or with alcohol and/or tranquilizers) represents the major substance of abuse. Factors which
underlie the epidemic abuse of cocaine include the following:

1. cocaine is easily available at all levels of society;
2. injection is not required for its use; and
3. cocaine is used freely by individuals in places of prominence and
   recognition; thus it is especially attractive to women as a 'first' drug of
   abuse.

Women addicted to cocaine are of particular interest to health care
workers concerned with the provision of obstetric care (see Chapter 5).
Unfortunately, whereas the literature on the interactions between opiate
abuse and pregnancy[1-4] is substantial, little data exists on cocaine abuse
and fertility-related matters.

Physicians providing primary health care to middle and upper classes of
society historically have refrained from confronting their patients with the
possibility of addiction. Over the years this 'protective' behavior has
tended to mask rather than deal with addictive problems, and therefore
should be abandoned, as each addicted individual within a given medical
practice is part of a larger system of epidemic proportions. Individual
health care providers must seek out drug-abusing behavior among their
patients rather than wait for patients to seek help after the fact.

THE PREGNANT ADDICT

General comments

Reported studies of pregnancy complicated by drug addiction occasionally fail to consider the lifestyle of substance abusers which is replete with
factors tending to complicate pregnancy. A partial listing of these factors
includes:

1. *The social environment of drug addicts.* The lifestyle of drug addicts is
   in a state of flux and frequently involves legal entanglements of a
   serious nature. In many instances the reliability of patient history
   reporting is low, and information obtained is open to question.
   Frequently the addict's nutritional status is less adequate than that of
   the general population and this circumstance may lead to profound
   effects on the developing fetus.
2. *Inadequate or no prenatal care.* Depending on the circumstances, as
   few as 25% of addicted pregnant women receive what is considered
   adequate maternity care[5].
3. *Variability of the patterns of drug abuse.* The type and availability of
   drugs fluctuates widely from city to city and within different areas of
   the same city. As marked changes in drug availability occur over
   relatively short periods of time, abuse of more than one drug is
   common – so much so that among known addicts it is unusual to
   encounter an individual whose abuse is limited to only one agent. The
   synergistic effects of the use of multiple drugs on the fetus are
   uncertain.

4. *Variable concentrations of active ingredients in street drugs.* The content of pharmacologically active agents in street drugs varies considerably from supplier to supplier and from day to day. It is generally agreed that many street drugs, especially heroin, contain a much lower quantity of the actual drug than they did 10 years ago.
5. *Adulterants.* Agents such as quinine, chalk, or sugar are universally found in street drugs. Not only is the concentration of active drug decreased in a given sample, but the effects of the adulterants are not always known.
6. *Unreliable information on drug effects.* Much of the data which form the basis of current medical opinion on drug effects has been obtained from less than ideal sources. Because simultaneous abuse of more than one drug is rampant, 'pure' study populations are virtually impossible to obtain. Even in well-controlled methadone maintenance programs the number of participants who 'chip' or use small quantities of illicit drugs during their pregnancy is high.

Superimposed upon the six factors noted above, pregnant women addicted to substances of abuse have psychological components to their addictive disorders which antedate the onset of their pregnancies and which remain after parturition. Unless the psychological as well as the physical components of addiction are treated concomitantly, the likelihood for relapse in one or the other area is great. In order to direct care to both aspects of the addictive process, it is of paramount importance to integrate health care providers from obstetric and psychiatric services into a cohesive team. Open communication within this team must be actively pursued to prevent manipulative patient behavior which may set individual team members at odds with each other.

Drugs of addictive power

Substances commonly abused during pregnancy are the same substances abused when women are not pregnant, with rare exceptions. The exceptions relate to the specific idiosyncrasies of women and their pregnancies. Thus, individual women may shy away from agents which accentuate their nausea or upset the gastrointestinal tract and replace these drugs with others which have the same general effect, absent the gastrointestinal upset upon early withdrawal. Table 3.1, taken from the National Institute of Drug Abuse Services Research Monograph Series, is a list of commonly abused agents, classified by site of action in the central nervous system[6].

Maternal complications

Medical

If the pregnant addict seeks prenatal care, she generally brings a host of medical complications with her[5,6]. Early diagnosis and prompt treatment of these problems are critical for their resolution. Recent data suggest that if pregnant addicts enroll early in a program designed to give comprehensive prenatal care and remain through parturition, most deliveries are

Table 3.1 Classification of drugs affecting the central nervous system

Effect	Trade name or synonym
I. Generalized effect	
A. *CNS depressants*	
Ethanol	Alcohol
Barbiturates	'Downers', 'barbs'
phenobarbital	
pentobarbital	Nembutal, 'yellow jackets'
secobarbital	Seconal, 'reds'
Nonbarbiturate sedatives–hypnotics	
glutethimide	Doriden
methaqualone	Quaalude, Sopor
ethchlorvynol	Placidyl
methyprylon	Noludar
hydroxyzine[1]	Atarax, Vistaril
meprobamate[1]	Equanil, Miltown
Hydantoins	
diphenylhydantoin (phenyltoin)	Dilantin
Benzodiazepines[1]	
chlordiazepoxide	Librium
diazepam	Valium
flurazepam	Dalmane
oxazepam	Serax
Anesthetics	
nitrous oxide	'Laughing gas'
halothane	Fluothane
Volatile solvents	
toluene	Toluol
naphtha	
benzine	
Cannabinoids (low dose)	
delta-9-tetrahydrocannabinol	THC
marijuana	'Grass'
hashish	'Hash'
B. *Stimulants*	
Amphetamines	'Uppers', 'speed'
amphetamine	Benzedrine
d-amphetamine	Dexedrine
methamphetamine	Methedrine, 'crystal'
Cocaine	
Caffeine	
Nicotine	
Phenmetrazine	Preludin
II. Localized effects	
A. *Affective (limbic) centers*	
1. Antipsychotic (depressant effect)	Major tranquilizers
Phenothiazines	
chlorpromazine	Thorazine
thioridazine	Mellaril
prochlorperazine	Compazine
trifluoperazine	Stelazine
fluphenazine	Prolixin
Butyrophenones	
haloperidol	Haldol
Thioxanthenes	
chloprothixene	Taractan
thiothixene	Navane

26

Table 3.1 Continued

2. Antidepressants	
(a) Tricyclics	
amitriptyline	Elavil
nortriptyline	Aventyl
imipramine	Tofranil
desipramine	Norpramin, Pertofrane
doxepin	Sinequan
(b) MAO inhibitors	
phenelzine	Nardil
3. Antimanics	
lithium	Lithonate
B. *Psychotogenic (hallucinogens)*	
lysergic acid diethylamide	LSD
dimethyltryptamine	DMT
mescaline	Cactus 'buttons'
psylocibin	'Magic mushrooms'
dimethoxyamphetamine	DOM, STP
phencyclidine	PCP
cannabinoids (large dose)	(see section IA of this table)
C. *Opioids*[2]	
1. Agonists	
morphine	
methylmorphine	Codeine
diacetyl morphine	Heroin
dihydromorphone	Dilaudid
camphorated opium tincture	Laudanum
methadone	Dolophine
propoxyphene	Darvon
L-alpha-acetyl methadol	LAAM
meperidine	Demerol
2. Antagonists	
naloxone	
naltrexone	Narcan
cyclazocine	
3. Mixed agonist–antagonists	
pentazocine	Talwin
nalorphine	Nalline
levalorphan	Lorfan

(From Reference 6)
[1] Frequently called minor tranquilizers
[2] Frequently termed "narcotics" or "opiates"

free of complications[4]. In contrast, maternal complications and problems in the newborn can be directly associated with a lack of prenatal care[3,7]. Table 3.2 lists common medical complications encountered in pregnant women addicted to opiates and especially heroin[6]. The relative frequencies of major complications in one reported study are cited in Table 3.3. Once again, however, these data were derived from a population of opiate abusers and may not hold true for a group of nonopiate-abusing pregnant women.

Table 3.2 Medical complications encountered in pregnant addicts

Anemia	Tetanus
Bacteremia	Tuberculosis
Cardiac disease, especially endocarditis	Urinary tract infections
Cellulitis	Cystitis
Poor dental hygiene	Urethritis
Diabetes mellitus	Pyelonephritis
Edema	Venereal disease
Hepatitis – acute and chronic	Condyloma acuminatum
Hypertension	Gonorrhea
Phlebitis	Herpes
Pneumonia	Syphilis
Septicemia	

(From Reference 6)

Table 3.3 Medical complications in addicted pregnant women

Complication	Incidence (%)
Anemia	61.9
Vaginitis	29.4
Positive serology	13.1
Hepatitis	9.4
Pyelonephritis	5.0
Acute gonorrheal vaginitis	4.4
Bartholin abscess	1.3
Pneumonia	0.6

(From Salerno, L. J. (1977) Prenatal care. In Rementeria, J. L. (ed.). *Drug Abuse in Pregnancy and Neonatal Effects*, p. 25 (St. Louis: Mosby) (from Reference 2).

Table 3.4 Obstetrical complications associated with heroin addiction

Abortion	Intrauterine death
Abruptio placentae	Intrauterine growth retardation
Amnionitis	Placental insufficiency
Breech presentation	Postpartum hemorrhage
Previous Cesarean section	Pre-eclampsia
Chorioamnionitis	Premature labor
Eclampsia	Premature rupture of membrane
Gestational diabetes	Septic thrombophlebitis

(From Reference 6)

Obstetric

The causal relations between heroin addiction and the obstetric complications listed in Table 3.4 are not always readily explained[6]. Some, such as chorioamnionitis, pre-eclampsia and/or eclampsia may be related to lack of prenatal care. Others, such as septic thrombophlebitis, may relate to infections resulting from the injection of abused substances. Still others, such as breech presentation and placental insuffuciency, are often difficult to explain even in the non-addicted patient. Table 3.5 shows obstetric complication rates in one study of heroin addicts compared with controls from the same institution.

Table 3.5 Comparison of obstetric complication rates in heroin addicts with those in total patient population

Complications	Incidence in addicts (%)	Overall incidence (%)
Abortion	14.0	12.3
Ectopic pregnancy	2.8	1.2
Birthweight less than 2500 g	24.3	4.8
Premature rupture of membranes	21.1	3.9
Toxemia	12.7	4.5
Placenta previa	1.7	0.7
Abruptio placentae	4.2	0.9
Malpresentation	9.3	3.5
Puerperal morbidity	11.9	2.9
Stillbirth	7.1	1.4

(From Pelosi *et al.* (1975). *Obstet. Gynecol.*, **45,** 512 and Rementeria *et al.* (1973). *Am. J. Obstet Gynecol.*, **116,** 1152)
(References 17 and 21)

It is generally thought that when the addicted mother is experiencing withdrawal symptoms, the fetus is experiencing some type of withdrawal symptomatology as well. The placenta of heroin-exposed infants commonly reveals meconium-stained histiocytes, suggesting that episodes of distress occurred during fetal life[8,9].

Between 18 and 50% of heroin addicts experience premature rupture of membranes[3,10]. The etiology of this amniorhexis is unknown. Even the lowest incidence rate (18%) exceeds the rate observed in a normal population. Possible causes include maternal infection with subsequent chorioamnionitis and uterine irritability associated with intermittent periods of narcotic withdrawal.

Data regarding stillbirths among infants born to heroin-addicted mothers must be interpreted with caution as a result of the multiplicity of confounding factors which may influence this specific outcome measure. In one study, published more than a decade ago, Rementeria[11] documented a five-fold to six-fold increase in the incidence of stillbirths in heroin-addicted women (71/1000).

THE MANAGEMENT OF DRUG ADDICTION IN PREGNANCY

Dole and Nyswander[12] first utilized methadone in 1965 for the clinical management of heroin addicts, and clinical trials of methadone use in pregnancy were reported in 1969[13]. The early initial enthusiasm for methadone substitution has been followed by a serious examination of the merits and drawbacks of using this medication in the treatment of the pregnant addict.

Six possible approaches to the management of the pregnant addict are listed and discussed below:

1. prenatal care and support with no attempt to alter the addiction pattern;
2. acute detoxification;
3. slow detoxification with methadone substitution and subsequent withdrawal;
4. methadone maintenance;
5. low-dose methadone maintenance combined with psychosocial counseling;
6. drug-free communities.

Supporting the patient prenatally without altering her addiction pattern implies the continuation of procurement of 'street' drugs and cyclic episodes of the 'highs' and 'lows' followed by withdrawal symptoms and occasional drug craving. Such behavior predictably is associated with higher risks for maternal and fetal complications.

When a pregnant woman undergoes acute withdrawal or detoxification ('cold turkey'), the fetus also experiences withdrawal. However, the fetus is less able to tolerate the insults of withdrawal than is its mother, and intrauterine death may result. Elective acute withdrawal or detoxification during pregnancy is almost never advised. Zuspan *et al.*[14] measured amino levels in amniotic fluid of addicted prenatal patients and found that significant increases in epinephrine and norepinephrine levels occurred in response to relatively mild reductions in methadone dosage. These investigators interpreted their findings as evidence of fetal distress and strongly recommended that detoxification not be attempted during pregnancy.

Some prenatal clinics advocate slow detoxification with substitution of methadone and subsequent withdrawal. However, this method of treatment fails to recognize two important points:

1. slow withdrawal also may be deleterious to the fetus; and
2. drug addiction is a more complex phenomenon than a mere physical dependence on drugs.

Unless the social and psychological aspects of addiction are considered concomitantly, it is unlikely that slow detoxification will be effective.

High doses (80 mg or more/day) can be used to effect a 'methadone blockade.' The rationale for this therapy is that tolerance develops at high dosages and the addict is less likely to get her usual 'high' if illicit heroin is also used. In contrast, low-dose methadone maintenance programs work on the premise that all opiates exert an adverse effect on the fetus. Accordingly, the pregnant addict is maintained on as low a dose as possible (5–40 mg/day).

In drug-free communities, patients are offered drug withdrawal, detoxification, and abstinence. Unless the addict is drug-free upon entry into the program, acute detoxification usually is mandated. This approach is often successful in the general population of drug addicts. In the pregnant addict, detoxification is discouraged for the reasons discussed above.

THE MEDICAL USE OF METHADONE

Since the pharmacologic actions of methadone are similar to those of heroin, the abuse potential is comparable. However, the maternal effects of methadone use may be different from those of heroin because methadone can be obtained legally and without charge. Although maintenance on the lowest possible dose is optimal, this dose must be sufficient to prevent supplementation with illicitly obtained heroin or methadone. If the maintenance dosage is too low, abuse with other drugs, including tranquilizers, sedatives or alcohol, may help alleviate withdrawal symptoms. As a result of problems obtaining an accurate history of the patient's heroin intake and the variability in the actual drug content of street heroin, the initial dose of methadone must be calculated with caution. Ideally, this dose should be based on a combination of physical examination and signs and symptoms of opiate withdrawal. A complete discussion of methadone maintenance in the pregnant narcotic addict can be found in Chapter 2.

MERITS AND DISADVANTAGES OF METHADONE USE

Many observers once considered methadone as a panacea. Unlike heroin, however, which is short-acting and pharmacologically available for only about 4 hours, methadone's activity spans approximately 24 hours. The therapeutic rationale for methadone use is to sustain the addict and hold withdrawal symptoms in abeyance. In pregnancy, the avoidance of the cyclic craving and withdrawal is especially important to the fetus. Methadone helps to establish a stabilized drug milieu for the fetus; theoretically, this stability should improve neonatal outcome. Critical evaluation of clinical experience with methadone use in pregnancy indicates that maternal complications are decreased and fetal outcome is improved[15]. Unfortunately, however, the neonatal course of infants whose mothers have used methadone is far from trouble-free. With regard to the infant, the merits of methadone use are generally confined to the prenatal period and its disadvantages to the neonatal period (Table 3.6). Many of the disadvantages cited in Table 3.6 are associated with high-dose (80 – 120 mg daily) methadone maintenance and can be eliminated by low-dose methadone maintenance (↑ 40 mg).

Published reports on the effect of methadone use in pregnancy span approximately 15 years and patterns of drug abuse have changed radically during this time. Confounding variables abound and may be so numerous and/or significant that no direct comparisons can be made between earlier reports and more recent observations. Unfortunately, polydrug use has increased markedly during this same time, and the vast majority of substances with potential for abuse have not been subjected to extensive study regarding their effects in pregnancy and on the neonate. In many instances available information is so scanty that any statements must be speculative. Extensive studies are needed to evaluate both the singular effects of these agents and their effects when combined with heroin or methadone. This is particularly true with regard to cocaine, the most popular substance of abuse today.

Table 3.6 Observations on methadone use in pregnancy

Advantages
Decreased incidence of low birthweight infants
Decreased incidence of prematurity
Decreased incidence of obstetric complications

Increased organ size and total cell number as compared with those of infants of untreated heroin-addicted mothers

Disadvantages
Increased incidence of low Apgar scores
Greater neonatal weight loss
Increased frequency, severity, and length of withdrawal symptoms as compared with those of infants of untreated heroin-addicted mothers
Increased incidence of convulsive seizures
Increased newborn serum bilirubin levels as compared with those of infants of untreated heroin-addicted mothers

Decreased visual orientation and following response in the infant
Initially depressed suck rates
Longer hospitalization and treatment of neonatal withdrawal symptoms

(From Reference 1)

Most participants in methadone maintenance programs do not use this drug exclusively. The problem of 'chipping' with heroin or other drugs adds a variable which is impossible to evaluate or control. Programs that routinely screen urines report that as many as 80% of their pregnant patients are 'dirty' at least once; a large percentage of them are 'dirty' on multiple occasions.

In spite of these problems, properly supervised methadone maintenance appears to exert a positive effect on pregnancy outcome. Serious questions have been raised, however, concerning neonatal effects and long-term effects of methadone on infant development (Table 3.6). In one such evaluation, not only is the intrauterine drug exposure important, but the effects of environment and the mother – child interaction must also be considered.

PRENATAL CARE

The team approach

Providing prenatal care to the pregnant addict is difficult. One estimate in 1975 suggested that 56% of all pregnant addicts received no prenatal care whatsoever[16]. It is not possible to state to what extent these figures have changed between 1975 and 1985. The lack of a reporting system which identifies and studies pregnant addicts nationally or locally precludes examination of data such as these.

Care of the pregnant addict should be based on the use of a multidisciplinary team with numerous support services at its disposal. The team should include representatives from at least three major areas:

1. an obstetrician capable of identifying and treating the medical problems encountered in the addicted female population or requesting referral when appropriate;
2. a psychologist or psychiatrist experienced in the care of drug-addicted patients and cognizant of the problems unique to them;
3. a specially trained nurse/social worker capable of offering guidance and support.

Supporting services should include the following at a minimum:

1. *financial services* to assist meeting basic needs;
2. *dietetic services* to provide information about proper nutrition;
3. *visiting nurse services* to aid in preparations for the newborn, and to make postpartum visits to supervise ongoing care of the infant;
4. *contraceptive counseling services* to offer information in the post-partum period.

Although members of the team may function individually, their efforts must be integrated and directed toward a common goal. Team members should meet regularly to review the status of all patients. The obstetrician should not direct the methadone dose or other aspects of drug management. Likewise, the psychologist/psychiatrist should be totally removed from obstetric decisions. Each member of the team should provide care commensurate with his/her area of expertise. This approach will negate any attempt of the addict to manipulate members of the team in order to secure favors, and uniform quality care is more likely to be provided.

Team members should remember that their goals extend beyond the pregnancy and should also be directed at long-term help and rehabilitation. To assist in this, the pregnant addict should see the same team members consistently. This will assist the patient in becoming acquainted with those responsible for her prenatal care and hopefully help to establish lines of trust and communication with them.

Prenatal obstetric care

Adequate care begins with a thorough medical evaluation and appropriate laboratory studies (Table 3.7). Maternal urine should be obtained at each visit and screened for the presence of illicit drugs. Routine parameters to evaluate fetal well-being should be employed.

Maternal or fetal infection must be aggressively treated. This is especially true for urinary tract infections, vaginitis, and venereal disease.

Tuberculosis, first identified during pregnancy by a positive skin test, should be evaluated by a chest X-ray with shielded abdomen. If a VDRL test is positive in low titer, the fluorescent treponemal antibody absorption (FTA-ABS) test should also be performed. Treatment should be undertaken only if the latter test is reactive and no prior treatment has been administered, as drug addiction itself may cause a weakly positive VDRL test. Intrauterine growth retardation should always be suspected although it is not always present, especially if patients receive early and adequate prenatal care[4].

Table 3.7 Initial routine laboratory tests

Complete blood count with indices	Serology (VDRL and FTA)
Urine:	Cervical–rectal culture for *N. gonorrheae*
Urinalysis – routine with microscopic	Cervical culture for chlamydia
Urine colony count and culture and sensitivity	Hepatitis-associated antigen (HAA)
Urine for drug screen	
	Cervical Pap smear
Chest X-ray or TB skin test	
	Blood type; Rh and indirect Coombs
Electrocardiogram	
	Alpha-fetoprotein if between 16 and 18 weeks gestation
	Ultrasound scan:
	1. For confirmation of pregnancy
Sickle prep when indicated	after 6 weeks gestation
	2. For biparietal diameter between
Rubella titer	20 and 30 weeks gestation

(From Reference 6)

A complete explanation for intrauterine fetal growth retardation is not provided solely by poor maternal nutritional habits. Some investigators have suggested the possibility that periodic episodes of heroin withdrawal might restrict fetal growth by reducing uterine or placental blood flow[9,17]. However, the organ and cellular growth pattern associated with fetal growth retardation in uteroplacental disorders is different from that observed in the offspring of heroin addicts. It seems possible that heroin has a direct effect on antenatal growth.

Ultrasound examinations to measure the biparietal diameter are advised. Ideally, these should be obtained between 20 and 26 weeks, 30 and 32 weeks, and 36 and 38 weeks of gestation to establish both gestational age and the fetal growth pattern. The growth-adjusted sonar age[18] is particularly valuable in this population, because accurate menstrual records generally are not kept and menstrual irregularity is common. Non-stress testing may be advisable weekly from the 36th week if IUGR is suspected.

Prenatal care should also include plans concerning delivery. Every possible effort should be made to effect delivery in an obstetric center equipped with a special care nursery to manage the neonate and any complications that may arise. The obstetric team should also assist the mother with the formation of concrete and rational plans for the care of her newborn upon discharge from the hospital.

Management of the pregnant addict in labor and postpartum

Management of the pregnant addict during labor is frequently complicated by the fact that the patient's drug habit is unknown to those caring for her. A high degree of suspicion is needed to identify these individuals as the addicted patient usually does not voluntarily reveal her addiction to the medical staff unless a crisis occurs. The presence of needle tracks or abscesses in the skin of a patient who arrives in labor with a history of no prenatal care should alert the physician to possible drug abuse.

It is common for an addict to remain at home until labor is well advanced, only to arrive at the hospital ready to deliver, usually 'high' on a last-minute drug fix to alleviate the pain of labor. Self-discharge against medical advice soon after delivery is a frequent occurrence, often within the first 24 hours. Should the patient remain longer, friends may help allay her drug craving and withdrawal by providing drugs. Table 3.8 is a summary of early and late signs and symptoms of maternal opiate withdrawal.

Table 3.8   Signs and symptoms of maternal withdrawal

Early	Late
Craving for drugs	Aching in bones and muscles
Thirst	Regurgitation
Anxiety	Diarrhea
Restlessness	Elevated blood pressure
Lacrimation	Hyperpyrexia
Tremors	Hyperventilation
Hot and cold flashes	Tachycardia
Diaphoresis	Abdominal girth
Nausea	Cramps
Yawning	Convulsions
Mydriosis	

Once the patient is in labor, the drug of choice to stabilize her condition and reverse the withdrawal process (if present) is methadone, given intramuscularly. If methadone is given orally, emesis may interfere with its absorption. Dosage should be based on the severity of the signs and symptoms. Table 3.9 presents guidelines for dose selection.

The therapeutic effect of intramuscular methadone is not achieved for 30–60 minutes. When withdrawal symptoms are severe, judicious use of a short-acting narcotic may be necessary. Recommended agents include morphine, meperidine (Demerol), methadone, and hydromorphine (Dilaudid). Pentazocine (Talwin) should *never* be administered, since this analgesic also acts as a potent narcotic antagonist and will precipitate an acute withdrawal reaction in an addicted individual[19]. Once withdrawal symptoms are under control (or if the patient is well maintained and not in withdrawal), the obstetrician is free to use whatever methods of anesthesia or analgesia are deemed necessary to provide pain relief for labor and delivery. In spite of their history of drug abuse and/or methadone maintenance, addicted parturients experience *real* pain with parturition. Withholding medications in the mistaken belief that these agents contribute to the addictive process is not necessary.

Table 3.9 Methadone doses in opiate withdrawal

Signs and symptoms	Initial methadone dose (mg)
Grade I	
Lacrimation, diaphoresis, yawning, restlessness, insomnia	5
Grade II	
Dilated pupils, muscle twitching, myalgia, arthalgia, abdominal pain	10
Grade III	
Tachycardia, hypertension, tachypnea, fever, anorexia, nausea, extreme restlessness	15
Grade IV	
Diarrhea, vomiting, dehydration, hyperglycemia, hypotension, curled-up position	20

(From Sultz, J. and Sevoy, E. (1975). Guidelines for management of hospitalized narcotic addicts. *Ann. Intern Med.*, **82**, 815)

Guidelines for managing labor and the postpartum period are the same as for the non-addicted patient. The infant, however, should be closely observed in the hospital for as long as necessary if drug abuse has been present antepartum. Methadone is excreted in breastmilk, and this should be noted when patients request to breastfeed their infants.

THE NORTHWESTERN MEMORIAL HOSPITAL EXPERIENCE

A special clinic for addicted pregnant women has been provided since 1976 at the Prentice Women's Hospital and Maternity Center of Northwestern Memorial Hospital. Started as a joint effort of the Departments of Psychiatry and Obstetrics and Gynecology, the clinic now has additional liaisons with the Departments of Pediatrics and Pharmacology. Numerous publications have resulted from our observations of these patients; most have been in the realm of pediatric follow-up and are discussed in Chapter 5. This section will summarize pertinent obstetric data. The demographic patient data were developed following review of patients delivered between April 1976 and October 1980[4]. The sonographic data were developed for this chapter from a review of records of patients delivered between 1980 and 1985.

The impact of intensive prenatal care on labor and delivery outcomes: demographic patterns and patient profile

Fifty-eight women were delivered of 62 infants. Two program participants returned to have a second child, and twin pregnancies occurred in two other women. The majority (70%) of the patients were under 25 years of age. White and Black patients were roughly equal in numbers. Half the patients had never been married; approximately one-quarter of the group stated they were currently married. The remainder were separated or divorced. Of particular interest was the educational background of these women: 41% had completed 12 or more years of formal education.

Antepartum obstetric history and risk factors

Whereas one-third of the patients were pregnant for the first time, more than half were expecting their first child. One or multiple abortions (spontaneous and induced) had been experienced in almost half of the patients. Since our patients were young, and abortion has been universally available since 1973, elements of criminality were not part of the history-taking process. Patients averaged almost nine prenatal visits. The various risk factors outlined in the standard Hollister obstetric history were not present in significant numbers. Although intrauterine growth retardation was occasionally suspected because of somewhat small uterine size for dates, subsequent ultrasound observations and delivery data did not confirm these clinical impressions. Smoking was popular (75%); alcohol consumption was not (20%).

Intrapartum and infant data

Tables 3.10 and 3.11 list important features of delivery and immediate neonatal data. Spontaneous vaginal delivery occurred in two-thirds of the cases; forceps were used in 20% of patients. Seven patients were delivered by Cesarean section for accepted obstetrical indications. The adjusted percentages of deliveries judged at term by weeks gestation was greater than 90%. When the weights of all infants were superimposed upon standard profiles for the US, the number of infants below the 50th percentile was slightly more than the number above it, but the difference was not remarkable. With regard to length, infants at term ranked almost equally above and below the 50th percentile. Four term infants were below the 10th percentile for head circumference and five were above the 90th percentile. Infants of drug-addicted mothers had a slight trend toward lower weights at term, and this trend carried to the length and head circumference. Table 3.12 compares average infant weights in our program with other recent published data. In stark contrast, the average weight of infants delivered to mothers actively addicted to heroin was 2393 g and the percentage of prematurity by weight was 52%[3].

Sonographic data

Figures 3.1 and 3.2 respectively depict the values of BPD and fetal weight at birth among 41 drug-addicted women delivered at Prentice Women's Hospital and Maternity Center between the years 1977 and May 1985. Analysis of the BPD data shows that the values tend to fall within the ranges expected in normal populations. In contrast, the fetal birthweights show that sufficient numbers fell below the 5th percentile as to suggest that asymmetric IUGR may have occurred in these infants. In other words, the head was spared at the expense of general growth. This tendency was not as marked in our earlier study of users[4] and conceivably may be related to polydrug abuse which was more common in this group of patients.

Table 3.10 The Northwestern University Dependence Program delivery data, 1976–80

	No.	*Percentage*
Gestational age (weeks):		
30–34	3	5.0
35–37	6	5.0
39–40	45	70.0
41–44	6	10.0
Birthweight (g):		
≤1500	1	1.6
1501–1999	1	1.6
2000–2499	11	17.7
2500–2999	24	38.4
3000–3499	12	19.4
≥3500	13	21.0

(From Reference 4)

Table 3.11 The Northwestern University Dependence Program infant data, 1976–80

	No.	*Percentage*
Apgar score at 1 min		
1–4	4	6.4
5–6	6	9.7
7–9	52	83.8
Apgar score at 5 min		
5–6	5	4.8
7–10	59	95.2
Medical complications:		
Respiratory distress syndrome	1	1.6
Meconium aspiration	1	1.6
Sepsis, culture negative	4	6.9
Other (jaundice)	5	8.1
None	51	82.2

(From Reference 4)

SUMMARY

This chapter summarizes recent literature on the obstetrical aspects of perinatal addiction. The experience at the Northwestern University Drug

Dependency Clinic is also reviewed and summarized. In our opinion, a multidisciplinary (obstetrical/psychological) team approach is required for optimal results.

Table 3.12 Mean weights of infants delivered of mothers in methadone programs

Author	Year	Mean weight (g)
Rosner et al.[4]	1982	2935
Stimmel and Adamsons[20]	1976	2933
Kendall et al.[21]	1976	2961
Newman et al.[22]	1976	2738*

* Mothers receiving 40 mg/d had infants with a mean of 2806g

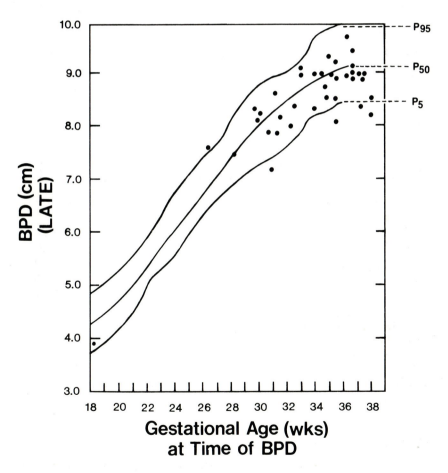

Figure 3.1

39

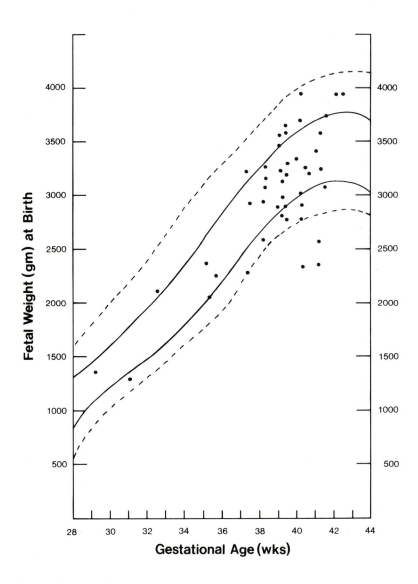

Figure 3.2

ACKNOWLEDGEMENT

The authors wish to thank Dr Rudy Sabbagha for assistance in analyzing sonographic data.

REFERENCES

1. Wager, G. and Keith, L. (1982). Drug addiction in pregnancy. In Depp, R., Eschenbach, D. A. and Sciarra, J. J. (eds) *Gynecology and Obstetrics*. Vol. 3, Chap. 31, pp. 1 – 10. (Philadelphia: Harper & Row)
2. Rementeria, J., Janakammal, S. and Hollander, M. (1975). Multiple births in drug-addicted women. *Am. J. Obstet. Gynecol.*, **122,** 958 – 60
3. Clark, D., Keith, L., Pildes, R. and Vargas, G. (1974). Drug-dependent obstetric patients. *J. Obstet. Gynecol. Nurs.*, **3,** 17 – 20
4. Rosner, M. A., Keith, L. and Chasnoff, I. (1982). The Northwestern University Drug Dependence Program: The impact of intensive prenatal care on labor and delivery outcomes. *Am. J. Obstet. Gynecol.*, **144,** 23 – 7
5. Connaughton, J., Reeser, D., Schut, J. and Finnegan, L. P. (1977). Perinatal addiction: outcome and management. *Am. J. Obstet. Gynecol.*, **129,** 679 – 86
6. Finnegan, L. P. (ed.) (1978). *Drug Dependence in Pregnancy: Clinical Management of Mother and Child*. National Institute on Drug Abuse, Services Research Monograph Series. (Rockville, MD: US Government Printing Office)
7. Moise, R., Reed, B. G. and Conell, C. (1981). Women in drug abuse treatment programs: Factors that influence retention at very early and later stages in two treatment modalities. A summary. *Int. J. Addict.*, **16,** 1295 – 1300
8. Naeye, R. L. (1965). Malnutrition: probable cause of fetal growth retardation. *Arch. Pathol.*, **79,** 284 – 91
9. Naeye, R., Blanc, W., Leblanc, W. and Khatamee, M. A. (1973). Fetal complications of maternal heroin addiction: abnormal growth, infections and episodes of stress. *J. Pediatr.*, **83,** 1055 – 61
10. Pelosi, M., Frattarola, M., Apuzzio, J., Langer, A., Hung, C. T., Oleske, J. M., Bai, J. and Harrigan, J. T. (1975). Pregnancy complicated by heroin addiction. *Gynecol. Obstet.*, **45,** 512 – 15
11. Rementeria, J. L. and Nunag, N. N. (1973). Narcotic withdrawal in pregnancy: stillbirth incidence with a case report. *Am. J. Obstet. Gynecol.*, **116,** 1152 – 6
12. Dole, V. P. and Nyswander, M. E. (1965). A medical treatment for diacetylmorphine (heroin) addiction: a clinical trial with methadone hydrochloride. *J. Am. Med. Assoc.*, **193,** 646 – 50
13. Wallach, R. C., Jerez, E. and Blinick, G. (1969). Pregnancy and prenatal function in narcotic addicts treated with methadone. *Am. J. Obstet. Gynecol.*, **105,** 1226 – 9
14. Zuspan, F. P., Gumpel, J. A., Mejia-Zelaya, A., Madden. J., Davis, R., Filer, M. and Tiamson, A. (1975). Fetal stress from methadone withdrawal. *Am. J. Obstet. Gynecol.*, **122,** 43 – 6
15. Finnegan, L., Schut, J. and Flor, J. (1977). Methadone maintenance and detoxification programs for the opiate-dependent woman during pregnancy. In Rementeria, J. L. (ed.) *Drug Abuse in Pregnancy and Neonatal Effects,* pp. 40 – 61. (St Louis: Mosby)
16. Abrams, C. A. L. (1975). Cytogenetic risks to the offspring of pregnant addicts. *Addict. Dis.*, **2,** 63 – 77
17. Wilson, G. S. (1975). Somatic growth effects of perinatal addiction. *Addict. Dis.*, **2,** 333 – 45
18. Sabbagha, R. E., Hughey, M. and Depp, R. (1978). Growth adjusted sonographic age: A simplified method. *Obstet. Gynecol.*, **51,** 383 – 6
19. Fultz, J. M. and Senay, E. C. (1975). Guidelines for the management of hospitalized narcotic addicts. *Ann. Intern. Med.*, **82,** 815 – 18
20. Stimmel, B., and Adamsons, K. (1976). Narcotic dependency in pregnancy. Methadone maintenance compared to use of street drugs. *J. Am. Med. Assoc.*, **235,** 1121 – 4
21. Kendall, S. R., Albin, S., Lowinson, J., Berle, B., Eidelman, A. I. and Gartner, L. M. (1976). Differential effects of maternal heroin and methadone use on birthweight. *Pediatrics*, **185,** 681 – 5
22. Newman, R. G., Bashkow, S. and Calko, D. (1975). Results of 313 consecutive live births of infants delivered to patients in the New York City methadone maintenance treatment program. *Am. J. Obstet. Gynecol.*, **121,** 233 – 7

4
A Comprehensive Treatment Model for Pregnant Chemical Users, Infants and Families

RALPH S. IENNARELLA, GAY M. CHISUM and JILL BIANCHI

INTRODUCTION

In 1976 the Chemical Dependence Program of Northwestern Memorial Hospital, with the assistance of Prentice Women's Hospital and Maternity Center, developed a program for expectant mothers, infants and their families. Perinatal Services offers comprehensive prenatal and post-partum care for the pregnant chemical user. This care is the product of a unique arrangement among chemical dependence, psychiatric, medical and educational services. In short, Perinatal Services recognizes the pregnant chemical user as a high-risk patient and provides a broad range of treatment, education and support for the expectant mother and her family.

At its inception Perinatal Services had a treatment staff consisting of a program coordinator, a nurse, a consulting obstetrician and pediatrician, and occasionally therapists from the Outpatient Chemical Dependence Program. The patient population ranged in number from 8 to 15 and was composed mainly of pregnant opiate abusers. Over the course of its development the program has been greatly expanded. Presently the treatment staff is composed of a program coordinator, a nurse, two clinical psychologists, a social worker, and two graduate students. Consultants to the program include two obstetricians, a pediatrician, two developmental psychologists, and a Lamaze instructor. The patient population ranges in number from 22 to 30 women in the prenatal and postpartum stages. The chemical-use problems include dependence on and abuse of opiates, stimulants, cannabis, sedative–hypnotics and hallucinogens.

The purpose of this paper is to present a comprehensive model for the psychotherapeutic treatment of the pregnant chemical user. This model recognizes the severity and pervasiveness of the phenomenon, appreciates the diverse and complex needs of the patient, and realizes the necessity of an approach which integrates the psychological, biological and social domains. It is hoped that this model will serve as a framework from which other programs may be developed.

REFERRALS AND DIAGNOSTIC EVALUATIONS

Women enter Perinatal Services from a variety of sources. A small number of women are self-referred. These are expectant mothers who are aware of the program's specialized services and request an evaluation. A larger number of women are referred to the program from within-hospital sources. These women are pregnant chemical users who come to the attention of a physician, nurse or social worker within the hospital complex. The staff member contacts Perinatal Services and schedules a consultation upon learning of or suspecting a chemical-use problem. A sizeable number of women are referred for treatment by outside sources. These sources typically consist of community hospitals, substance abuse programs, and various governmental agencies (e.g. the Department of Alcohol and Substance Abuse). The patient contacts the program and schedules an evaluation.

During the evaluation session the patient undergoes a thorough and systematic diagnostic interview to determine the extent and nature of the chemical-use problem. The core of the evaluation is a screening instrument which is used at Northwestern Memorial Hospital's Chemical Dependence Program[1]. A comprehensive alcohol and drug history is taken, in conjunction with a medical history, a mental status examination and an assessment of the patient's social support system. While this traditional type of screening provides essential information, the evaluation is tailored to assess the unique characteristics and circumstances of the pregnant chemical user.

Particular attention is placed on the type and quantity of drugs consumed during each month of the pregnancy, beginning with the month prior to the last menstrual period. Outlining the patient's chemical use during pregnancy in this way provides a detailed account of chemical exposure during the different stages of fetal development. Additionally, a month-by-month breakdown of the chemical use allows an assessment of fetal activity as a variation of the type and quantity of drug consumed. This analysis of fetal activity provides the expectant mother with a concrete method for better appreciating how chemical use affects her unborn child.

The medical history generally taken with chemical dependence patients is broadened to include areas specifically related to pregnancy. Thus the patient is questioned about her prenatal care and the extent to which the obstetrician knows about her chemical use. Previous pregnancies are reviewed with respect to chemical use, complications with labor and delivery, and whether the pregnancies were carried to full term. The current pregnancy is carefully screened for possible signs of complications, such as cramping, spotting, bleeding and weight loss. This entire line of questioning greatly aids the evaluator's decision-making process with respect to the patient's needed level of care.

An assessment of the patient's social support system is conducted in relation to both the chemical use and the pregnancy. Important lines of investigation would include whether the pregnancy was planned, how the father is responding to the pregnancy, and how the patient is responding to the father's reaction. Other areas that need exploration are the likelihood of abortion and adoption, the father's chemical use, his reaction to the patient's interest in treatment, and the availability of others to assist with child care. Assessing the social support system in this manner has much prognostic value with respect to the patient's chances for following through with treatment recommendations.

Based upon the findings of the evaluation, the patient begins treatment either on an inpatient or outpatient basis.

METHADONE TREATMENT

Approximately half of the expectant mothers presenting to Perinatal Services are dependent on opioids. Although there is some controversy as to whether an attempt should be made to withdraw opioids from the mother during pregnancy, an abrupt cessation of opioids is clearly hazardous and may precipitate a number of obstetric complications, particularly spontaneous abortion or premature labor[2]. Consequently, pregnant women who are dependent on opioids are placed on methadone maintenance. Methadone is therapeutically advantageous because it is long-acting, effective orally, relatively inexpensive, and has few known side-effects[3]. As part of the treatment, random urine samples are obtained regularly and screened for illicit drug use.

The initial daily dosage of methadone varies among women in the program. The dosage is decreased to the lowest level which prevents withdrawal and craving. Following the recommendations of Finnegan[4], methadone levels are not usually decreased during the first and third trimesters due to risks of spontaneous abortion and premature delivery. During the past 3 years, however, Perinatal Services has begun to investigate methadone withdrawal in the second trimester with continuation of the detoxification through the third trimester. This has been conducted in both inpatient and outpatient settings. Methadone detoxification has been deemed appropriate when the patient demonstrates a trusting relationship with her therapist, is medically stable, has no major psychiatric disturbance, and has a stable lifestyle with an available support system.

ACUTE HOSPITAL CARE

Acute Hospital Services is a 21-day inpatient program utilized when the use of chemicals dominates the expectant mother's life, physical complications are present, the risk of withdrawal is high, and isolation from others exacerbates a limited ability to manage the responsibilities of daily living. In addition to use as a form of crisis intervention, hospital care is instituted by Perinatal Services as a matter of course when a patient first enters treatment at 7 or more months of pregnancy. This policy was developed in response to difficulties in engaging these women in treatment during the last trimester of pregnancy. The Acute Hospital Services program is designed to accomplish two principal goals. First, a safe and stable environment is provided for the expectant mother. This environment allows for the evaluation, management and monitoring of withdrawal from any chemical or combination of chemicals. The hospital setting also provides an environment where medical complications can be assessed, treated and stabilized. The second goal of Acute Hospital Services is to provide the pregnant woman with a structured milieu. Within this milieu the patient is encouraged to begin a change in lifestyle, and to look to other people for shared experiences, support and guidance.

An integral part of the acute care phase is the patient's linkage to appropriate resources at the completion of the inpatient stay. With respect to the pregnant chemical user, a referral to Perinatal Services for outpatient treatment is understood from the outset. What is novel about this is the arrangement between Acute Hospital Services and Perinatal Services for the patient's early involvement with the latter program. Early in the patient's hospitalization she begins to participate in prescribed treatment components of Perinatal Services. This conjoint involvement in two treatment programs demands a good deal of planning and coordination.

Shortly after a patient's admission to the hospital unit, an inpatient treatment plan is developed by a multidisciplinary team that includes a representative from Perinatal Services. This representative is the patient's assigned outpatient therapist. As part of the inpatient treatment plan, the team decides in which perinatal components the patient will participate. This plan is then implemented, with the two treatment programs consulting frequently to ensure that the treatment does not overwhelm the patient and the various objectives do not conflict with one another.

Clinical experience has shown that the advantages of coordinating and implementing Acute Hospital Services and Perinatal Services conjointly are many. While in the hospital the patient begins to develop an alliance and treatment relationship with Perinatal Services overall and the outpatient therapist in particular. This helps to increase the likelihood that the patient will follow through with outpatient treatment beyond the completion of the inpatient stay. In addition, conjoint treatment by both programs provides a holistic approach to the acute and long-term needs of the patient, both in terms of the pregnancy and the chemical-use problem.

The situation often arises where a patient initially begins treatment as an outpatient and subsequently needs hospitalization. Here, too, the outpatient therapist meets with the inpatient team so that a treatment plan includes the patient's continued involvement in outpatient services while hospitalized. The involvement can be extensive and wide-ranging, due to the multifaceted design of Perinatal Services.

PERINATAL SERVICES

Treatment for the pregnant chemical user is a long-term process which depends on the patient assuming responsibility for herself and her family, without the use of chemicals. Many of the women coming into the program have not developed the strengths and skills necessary for this. Consequently, an active and productive lifestyle is contingent not only upon abstinence, but also upon the development of basic skills and abilities. Perinatal Services is a comprehensive treatment program designed to meet the many needs of the recovering, pregnant chemical user.

Services within the program are differentiated according to whether a patient is at the prenatal or postpartum stage of delivery. While certain modes of treatment are ongoing, others are added, eliminated and adapted as a woman passes from pregnancy to parenthood.

Prenatal treatment

This treatment package has been developed for women who are experiencing the vast physical and psychological changes of pregnancy. The package consists of individual psychotherapy, group therapy, prenatal education class, Lamaze training and obstetrics clinic.

Individual psychotherapy is a required component of treatment for women in Perinatal Services. The consistency, reliability, and intimacy which characterizes the therapeutic relationship provides a nexus for the broad range of treatments in which the patient will be engaged. Though the individual therapy is conducted and managed differently from one therapist to another, there is a general program philosophy which characterizes this treatment mode. This type of treatment approach has been described by Khantzian[5] and is consistent with the substantial body of knowledge that has accumulated on the psychological factors related to serious chemical use.

A sizeable pool of clinical data and research findings indicates that one of the major motivations for chemical use is the seeking of immediate gratification of primitive, dependent needs in a state in which the longing for others is lost in an experience of narcissistic pleasure[6]. Considerable dysphoria may be experienced around issues of loneliness, helplessness and feeling unloved and abandoned. Yet there is a reluctance or inability to seek satisfaction in normal interpersonal relationships. The chemical use replaces interpersonal relationships as a primary source of achieving satisfaction and pleasure. This seems clearly related to the profound emotional deprivation that occurs early in the chemical user's life. In line with the above, the therapist attempts to work with the patient to gain control over the chemical use and the destructive behavior often associated with it. The patient's tendencies to engage in the extremes of indulgence and self-denial are identified, and fears of involving oneself with others are explored. The patient's current lifestyle is seen to be intimately tied to her childhood experiences and her familial relationships. The therapist helps the patient to understand her issues with parenthood as they relate to the quality of nurturance she received during childhood and the parental role models to which she was exposed. The therapist also actively points out the patient's inability or disinclination to recognize the danger and risk in her lifestyle. In short, the individual treatment focuses squarely on the chemical-use problem and the underlying psychopathology within the context of pregnancy and parenthood.

Group therapy is strongly recommended to women in the program. A patient is generally referred for group treatment once she has stabilized within her individual treatment. The treatment is conceptualized and approached according to the theoretical framework provided by Yalom[7]. Thus the group permits a sharing of experiences and feelings and offers the women a chance to understand that they are not unique in their problems and attempted solutions. Because of painful life situations these women often experience intense feelings of anxiety, guilt, shame, fear and depression. Chemical users often lack adequate psychological resources to modulate and contain these painful affects[8]. They are frequently flooded by painful and dysphoric affect and seek pleasure via some immediate, isolated and temporary solution. The essential aims of the group treatment are the support of one's peers and the development of improved relationships, whereby the women can begin to seek and gain pleasure in the normal interpersonal experiences of everyday life. Conflicts and feelings relating to pregnancy, chemical use, parenting and varying personal needs and wishes are actively addressed.

Although couples, marital and family treatments are not specifically built into the structure of Perinatal Services, these treatment modalities are strongly recommended to patients and their families. Generally, the patient's individual therapist assesses the need for these modalities and then makes the necessary referral. Up to this time there has been limited success in engaging the natural father and significant others in treatment. In fact, family members have often attempted to sabotage the patient's treatment, sometimes resulting in premature termination from the program.

The prenatal education class is a 16-session series which includes lectures, films, demonstrations, reading materials and discussions. The class focuses on three main topics: addiction and the addictive process, the physical and psychological ramifications of pregnancy, and the fetal effects of chemical use. With respect to the latter topic, for example, the women learn how their chemical use affects the intrauterine environment, interferes with normal fetal development, and influences neonatal behavior. The women are also taught to recognize the signs and symptoms of withdrawal which their infants will experience post-delivery. Strategies and techniques are provided for consoling and soothing the infant during the withdrawal phase. In addition, the risk of sudden infant death syndrome (SIDS) is addressed, and the need for training in cardiopulmonary resuscitation (CPR) is strongly encouraged. Although CPR classes are not provided by the program, arrangements are made with outside agencies. Attention is also given to family relations, and how these interface with pregnancy, parenthood and chemical use. Particular attention is given to the baby's father and his involvement.

Each patient has the option of attending eight Lamaze classes. Patients are encouraged to bring their mates or significant others to the classes. The Lamaze training is directed primarily towards providing patients with a means of managing the anxiety and pain associated with labor and delivery. The hope is that this training will decrease the possibility of illicit drug use prior to labor and delivery[9].

Finally, Perinatal Services has developed a specialized, high-risk obstetrics clinic for the pregnant chemical user. The value of intensive prenatal care for labor and delivery has been indicated by Rosner et al[10]. The obstetrics clinic is staffed by two obstetricians and a nurse, who meet with the patients according to their individual needs. The obstetrical care routinely includes general laboratory and blood tests, up to four ultrasounds, and consultation with a nutritionist. Specialized care includes evaluation and treatment for hepatitis, chlamydia and other sexually transmitted diseases. The clinic team also works to reassure patients in regard to their fears and anxieties about pregnancy and childbirth. By having the same team following the patients, the women have an opportunity to become familiar with the doctors and nurse and develop a sense of trust in them.

Postpartum treatment

After a woman delivers, she and her infant begin participation in a treatment program designed to facilitate normal child development and an optimal parent–child relationship. Babysitting services are provided to allow regular attendance. The individual and group treatments, which were initiated during the prenatal phase, are maintained as the principal forms of psychotherapy. The prenatal education class is replaced by a postpartum series which focuses on parenting and child development. With the inclusion of a pediatric clinic, a developmental clinic, and a mother–infant therapy group, the mother and her infant are provided a full range of services.

As the individual psychotherapy progresses with the patient's advancement from the prenatal to the postpartum stage, conflicts relating to parenthood and chemical use emerge. The therapist's availability as a stable figure can be particularly meaningful to the patient, in light of the therapist's earlier involvement with the pregnancy, labor and delivery. The therapist's intimate knowledge of, and involvement with, the patient's prenatal care offers a context to the patient for seeing the therapist as available, concerned and understanding.

The patient continues her participation in group treatment during the postpartum stage. The composition of the group thus includes women at the prenatal and postpartum stages. The inclusion of both expectant and new mothers has proved beneficial, particularly in terms of the patients' gaining needed support. Postpartum women are often able to offer the prenatal women reassurance regarding their anxieties about labor and delivery. Prenatal women who are conscientiously attempting to refrain from using chemicals can support and reinforce the abstinence of women who are prone to return to chemical use once they have delivered. The mix of patients within the group creates a vitality which makes the group experience meaningful and relevant.

The postpartum education class is a 50-session series which utilizes the same format as the prenatal class. Chemical-use issues are a focus throughout the class and are addressed with respect to four main topics: parenting and child development, discipline and child abuse, women's issues, and employment. Overall, the class stresses the role of the parent as being a model for the child's behavior. Throughout, the effects of chemical use on the ability to parent are emphasized. This notion is especially developed in relation to normal child development and behavior. The mothers are provided with techniques for teaching their children new behaviors and appropriately disciplining unacceptable ones. While the emphasis is placed upon the woman's role as parent, the class also extends beyond this to include such issues as intimacy, sexuality, employment and day care.

The pediatric clinic was designed specifically for infants and children born to mothers who used chemicals during their pregnancies. The clinic is headed by a pediatrician whose expertise includes the recognition and management of infants and children exposed to chemicals *in utero*[11]. Infants and children are seen on an individual basis as needed. The pediatrics clinic provides total well-baby care, including regular checkups and immunizations. All of the newborns are closely observed for signs of acute and prolonged withdrawal[12,13]. Pediatric clinic is also a means by which the mothers obtain guidance and support, particularly in terms of acknowledging and accepting the effects of their chemical use on their infants.

Neonatal developmental testing and follow-up is provided on an extensive level through Northwestern Memorial Hospital's Developmental Clinic. Two pediatric developmental psychologists from this clinic serve as consultants to Perinatal Services. Within 72 hours of life, all infants in the program are evaluated with the Brazelton Neonatal Behavioral Assessment Scale[14]. Thereafter, each infant is tested every 3 months during the first year, every 6 months through age 4 years, and every 12 months during succeeding years. Along with the Brazelton, a battery of age-appropriate developmental tests is utilized. Mother – infant interactions are also observed and evaluated. The neonate's development is thus carefully followed, and this information is continuously shared with the parents and the perinatal staff. The essential aim of this information is to provide for early detection of developmental difficulties and to suggest effective intervention strategies and techniques.

The mother–infant group was originated in response to the developmental difficulties evidenced by infants during the acute and prolonged phases of chemical withdrawal. An infant in the throes of withdrawal is difficult to console, thereby leading the mother to feel anxious and inadequate. The mother may withdraw from the infant out of deep frustration. The result is a dysfunctional mother – infant relationship which exacerbates existing developmental difficulties and promotes the unfolding of new ones[15]. The mother–infant group teaches mothers effective means of caring for their infants during the withdrawal phase. More broadly, the group attempts to focus on developmental issues and offers support and education. The women and their babies meet on a weekly basis, which enables the therapist and women to more effectively observe the babies' behavior and the mothers' relationships with their infants. It is in the mother – infant group where much of the information gleaned from the pediatric and developmental clinics is integrated and utilized to improve mother – infant interactions.

FUTURE DIRECTIONS

Since the program first began, Perinatal Services has developed and expanded in accordance with patients' needs. This continues to be the main impetus behind program development. There are currently a number of services which are being planned.

As noted above, Perinatal Services has had limited success in engaging family members in treatment. This has been especially so with respect to the fathers of the babies. Most of these fathers appear to be heavy chemical users and regard the program as a threat. A workshop for these fathers has been designed in an attempt to encourage them to become more involved with the mother's treatment and the child's care. A time-limited (i.e. four sessions) workshop which focuses on education, instruction and discussion will hopefully be perceived as relatively nonthreatening.

The workshop will address three main topics: the physical and psychological changes of pregnancy, delivery and the postpartum period; the fetal effects of alcohol and drug use; the need for fathers to be more involved with child care. Since these areas will be targeted, and not the fathers' own chemical use, it is expected the men would more likely accept this invitation from the program. During their participation in the workshop the fathers will become acquainted with the range of services offered through the program. It is hoped that through this experience the fathers will be more supportive of their mate's treatment, if not more directly involved.

Another project under development concerns babysitting services. Presently a professional babysitter assumes responsibility for child care when mothers are involved in some component of their treatment which does not include the child. Plans are under way for turning over the child care to expectant mothers in the program, who would care for the infants and children under the supervision of a trained professional. This would provide expectant mothers an opportunity to observe and gain experience with infants who are evidencing signs of acute withdrawal.

Finally, it has become obvious that a number of women entering Perinatal Services need a form of residential treatment which would allow an extended period of time during which crucial changes in living arrangements could be made. A residential program would provide women with temporary housing, vocational counseling and a supportive treatment environment. Moreover, children could reside with their mothers, thereby allowing the treatment to occur without disrupting the mother – child relationship. Perinatal Services is exploring the possibility of instituting such a residential treatment program.

REFERENCES

1. Haller-Johnson, D., Kinney, C. and Schnoll, S. H. (1984). Initiating outpatient withdrawal for the chemically dependent patient. *Family Commun. Health,* **8,** 1 – 15
2. MacGillivray, I. and Hall, H. (1980). Obstetric and gynaecological disorders. In Avery, G. S. (ed.) *Drug Treatment.* (New York: Adis Press)
3. Cohen, S. (1981). *The Substance Abuse Problems.* (New York: Haworth Press)
4. Finnegan, L. P. (1975). Narcotic dependence in pregnancy. *J. Psychedelic Drugs*, **7,** 304 – 6
5. Khantzian, E. J. (1978). The ego, the self, and opiate addiction: theoretical and treatment considerations. *Int. Rev. Psychoanal.*, **5,** 189 – 98
6. Blatt, S. J., McDonald, C., Sugarman, A. and Wilber, C. (1984). Psycho-dynamic theories of opiate addiction: new directions for research. *Clin. Psychol. Rev.*, **4,** 159 – 89
7. Yalom, I. (1970). *The Theory and Practice of Group Psychotherapy.* (New York: Basic Books)
8. Wurmser, L. (1978). *The Hidden Dimension.* (New York: Jason Aronson)
9. Ostrea, E., Chavez, C. and Stryker, J. (1978). *The Care of The Drug Dependent Woman and Her Infant.* (Michigan Department of Public Health)
10. Rosner, M. A., Keith, L. and Chasnoff, I. J. (1982). The impact of intensive prenatal care on labor and delivery outcomes. *Am. J. Obstet. Gynecol.*, **144,** 23 – 7
11. Chasnoff, I. J., Hatcher, R. and Burns, W. J. (1982). Polydrug- and methadone-addicted newborns: a continuum of impairment? *Pediatrics*, **70,** 210 – 13
12. Chasnoff, I. J., Hatcher, R. and Burns, W. J. (1980). Early growth patterns of methadone-addicted infants. *Am. J. Dis. Child.*, **134,** 1049 – 51
13. Chasnoff, I. J. and Burns, W. J. (1984). The Moro reaction: a scoring system for neonatal narcotic withdrawal. *Devel. Med. Clin. Neurol.*, **26,** 484 – 9
14. Brazelton, T. B. (1976). *Neonatal Behavioral Assessment Scale.* (Philadelphia: Spastics International Medical Publications)
15. Greenberg, S. I. (1981). *Psychopathology and Adaptation in Infancy and Early Childhood.* (New York: International Universities Press)

5
Perinatal Addiction: Consequences of Intrauterine Exposure to Opiate and Nonopiate Drugs

IRA J. CHASNOFF

> The seed when attached must be nourished, and takes food from the substance containing blood and pneuma which is brought to it. But in drunkenness and indigestion all vapor is spoilt and the pneuma too is rendered turbid. Therefore, danger arises, lest by reason of the bad material contributed, the seed too changes for the worse. Furthermore, the satiety due to heavy drinking hinders the attachment to the uterus.
>
> Soranus of Ephesus (Rome, first or second century, AD)

The problems of drug abuse during pregnancy have been with us since antiquity. Soranus' caution against the use of alcohol during pregnancy and the Biblical injunction against newlyweds' imbibing lest they injure the unborn child (Judges 13:7) serve as early warnings on the danger of substance abuse during pregnancy. In 1973, with the modern description of the fetal alcohol syndrome by Jones et al[1]., public attention in the United States was directed toward the possible teratogenic effects of recreational drugs consumed during pregnancy. Around this time, also, descriptions of withdrawal suffered by neonates exposed *in utero* to narcotics (heroin or methadone)[2] emphasized the need for further study of the behavioral and neurological effects of drugs on the developing fetus and child.

It is now widely recognized that women of childbearing age are regular users of licit and illicit drugs[3], and in the past decade the list of substances known to affect the unborn child has broadened. Additionally, our concept of teratology has changed in that we now recognize that although most drugs of use and abuse do not produce congenital malformations, there are definite behavioral and neurological effects that impair the neonate's, infant's and child's development. It is the purpose of this paper to review the characteristics of withdrawal patterns in neonates exposed to various substances during gestation and to outline methods of management, treatment and long-term evaluation of these children. Since alcohol and marijuana have a frequent role in polydrug abuse, serving as secondary as well as primary drugs of abuse, each of these substances will be additionally discussed in separate chapters.

NEONATAL ABSTINENCE SYNDROME

Early studies of infants delivered to heroin-using mothers showed that these infants had a higher rate of perinatal morbidity and mortality than infants in the general population[4,5]. Common problems associated with heroin use during pregnancy were first-trimester spontaneous abortions, premature delivery, neonatal meconium aspiration syndrome, maternal/neonatal infections including venereal diseases, and severe neonatal withdrawal. Attempts to provide better control of these pregnancies were anchored in methadone maintenance programs in which pregnant women attended prenatal obstetric clinics and received daily methadone to replace their use of street heroin. The initial methadone maintenance programs were successful in that the more consistent medical and nutritional care provided for these women resulted in improved pregnancy outcome[6]. However, the high doses of methadone (80–120 mg per day) produced a more severe and prolonged period of abstinence for the newborn as compared to the patterns of withdrawal for infants exposed to heroin[7].

Table 5.1 Signs and symptoms of neonatal abstinence syndrome

Tremors	Nasal stuffiness
Restlessness	Rapid respirations
Hyperactive reflexes	Frequent yawning
Vomiting, diarrhea	Sweating
Increased muscle tone	Excoriation of knees, elbows
High-pitched cry	Mottling of skin
Sneezing	Fever
Voracious sucking	Lacrimation
Sleeplessness	Seizures
Stretching	

It was during this period of time that a complete description of the neonatal abstinence syndrome was reported by Finnegan et al.[2]. The most common features of the neonatal abstinence syndrome as outlined in Table 5.1 mimicked aspects of an adult withdrawing from narcotics. Most significant for the neonate were the high-pitched cry, sweating, tremulousness, excoriation of the extremities and gastrointestinal upset. In an effort to reduce the degree of withdrawal for the newborn, low-dose methadone maintenance programs for pregnant women were developed[6], and it is now the general recommendation to maintain a pregnant woman on as low a dose of methadone as possible. A full description of low-dose methadone maintenance can be found in Chapter 1.

Symptoms of neonatal withdrawal from narcotics are usually present at birth but may not reach a peak until 3–4 days of life[2,8,9]. Onset of withdrawal depends, however, on many factors, and symptoms may not appear until 10–14 days after birth. This delay in onset of withdrawal is especially true for some nonopiate drugs, such as phenobarbital[10]. Withdrawal from opiates persists in a subacute form for 4 – 6 months after birth, with a peak in symptoms at around 6 weeks of age[11]. Neurologic effects due to intrauterine opiate exposure have been noted with abnormalities of the Moro reaction documented through as late as 7–8 months of age[12].

Abstinence symptoms in the neonate exposed to nonopiate drugs *in utero* have been described for phenobarbital[10], secobarbital[13], diazepam[14], chlordiazepoxide[15] and alcohol[16]. Although withdrawal from these substances does not appear to result in as severe a syndrome of abstinence as withdrawal from narcotics, the newborn does exhibit the irritability, restlessness, poor feeding, crying and impaired neurobehavioral abilities that are characteristic of the neonatal abstinence syndrome[17].

TREATMENT OF NEONATAL ABSTINENCE

Treatment of the neonate for withdrawal should be supportive, since pharmacologic therapy can prolong hospitalization and exposes the infant to additional agents which often are not necessary. Mothers of infants exposed *in utero* to substances which produce withdrawal should be taught to swaddle the infant closely and tightly in a blanket. Use of a pacifier also soothes the infant's irritability and relieves the increased sucking urge experienced by the withdrawing infant. Frequent small feedings are better tolerated and should provide 150–250 cal/kg per 24 hours for proper growth of the infant undergoing abstinence[18].

Pharmacologic therapy should be based on conclusions developed through the use of one of the various abstinence scoring methods[19,20]. Excessive weight loss or dehydration due to vomiting and diarrhea, inability of the infant to feed or sleep, fever unrelated to infection, or seizures are the most common clinical indications for drug treatment. Other causes for these symptoms, such as infection, metabolic abnormalities (hypoglycemia, hypocalcemia), hyperthyroidism, central nervous system hemorrhage and birth anoxia should be considered before therapy is begun.

Most information regarding the pharmacologic treatment of neonatal abstinence is based on experience derived from the therapy of narcotic withdrawal. There is little research information regarding pharmacologic therapy of the infant who has been exposed *in utero* to nonopiate drugs. Three agents have served as the basis for pharmacologic therapy of neonatal withdrawal from narcotics: paregoric (anhydrous morphine, 0.4 mg/ml), diazepam and phenobarbital.

The major advantage of paregoric is the ease of administration. In addition, infants treated with paregoric have improved and more efficient sucking behavior, and exhibit better weight gain, than infants treated with diazepam or phenobarbital[21]. The dose of paregoric administered to an infant for treatment of abstinence symptoms ranges from 0.2 to 0.5 ml per dose every 3–4 hours until the symptoms of withdrawal are controlled. A neonatal abstinence score is helpful in titrating the dose, and the medication should be tapered off after symptoms have been stabilized for 4 – 5 days.

A major concern regarding the use of opiate preparations in neonates is the marked respiratory depressant effect. Morphine doses of 0.1 mg/kg have been reported to cause respiratory cessation in nonnarcotic-habituated infants, although infants manifesting narcotic withdrawal would be more tolerant of this dose[22].

Diazepam, in a dosage of 1–2 mg every 8 hours, rapidly suppresses narcotic withdrawal symptoms in the neonate. However, the newborn infant has a limited capacity to metabolize diazepam and total elimination may take up to 1 month[23]. Parenteral diazepam contains benzyl alcohol and sodium benzoate, which may displace bilirubin for conjugation and excretion; therefore, diazepam should not be used in an icteric or premature infant[24]. Use of diazepam can be associated with depression of the neonatal sucking reflex, and late-onset seizures have occurred in neonates after cessation of treatment with diazepam[25].

Phenobarbital will quieten the infant with neonatal withdrawal, but it does little for the gastrointestinal symptoms. Large doses of phenobarbital exert a marked sedative effect on the central nervous system of the infant and impair sucking. A neonatal loading dose of 16 mg/kg per 24 hours of phenobarbital to produce blood levels of 20 – 30 fg/ml with maintenance doses of 2 – 8 mg/kg per 24 hours to keep the medication at a therapeutic blood level has been reported to control withdrawal symptoms in term neonates[26]. Blood levels of phenobarbital should be followed closely and adjusted according to the infant's symptoms and the abstinence score results. After the infant's symptoms have stabilized, the daily dose of phenobarbital should be decreased to allow the drug level to decrease by 10 – 20% per day.

Pharmacologic therapy of infants with symptoms of abstinence due to exposure to nonopiate drugs is usually not necessary, since these infants rarely require any more than supportive therapy. If an infant in this situation should require pharmacologic intervention, phenobarbital, given in the same manner as for opiate withdrawal described above, would be the medication of choice.

EVALUATION OF THE NEONATE AND INFANT

Evaluation of the infant delivered to a substance-abusing mother requires a multifaceted approach, coordinated by a physician and nursing staff familiar with the problems associated with neonatal abstinence. A record of feeding patterns for the child should be kept and daily weights recorded. An organized assessment scale for neonatal withdrawal should be kept at the bedside to ensure objective evaluation of the level of abstinence symptoms undergone by the infant[19,20].

Formal evaluation of the neonate's neurologic status has most frequently entailed the use of the Brazelton Neonatal Behavioral Assessment Scale (BNBAS)[27]. This scale is a multi-item scale developed to assess the neurobehavioral status of infants less than 28 days of age. Approximately half the scale is an evaluation of neonatal reflexes and half the scale is an evaluation of behavioral items such as interactive abilities and state organization. In our program at Northwestern University the infants are evaluated at 3 days and again at 4 weeks of age in a quiet, dimly lit room. Information gained from the BNBAS is used to complement the clinical evaluation of the infants and to instruct each mother in specific areas of deficiencies which might be present in her particular infant.

Infants should be followed weekly during the first month of life, with specific attention given to growth and development, level of withdrawal and adequacy of maternal–infant interaction. Abnormalities in any of these areas should be cause for concern and intervention on the part of the medical personnel evaluating mother and child. If the infant is doing relatively well at this point, evaluations can be reduced to every 2–4 weeks, depending on the clinical impression of the examiner. Monthly exams should continue at least through 6 months of age, by which time subacute withdrawal usually abates[11]. Exams every 3 months are usually adequate after this, and should continue through 2 years of age followed by every 6 months exams through 4 years of age, then once a year evaluations for as long as possible. Schedules can be adjusted, certainly, according to the facilities and personnel available for each program.

THE PERINATAL SERVICES PROJECT OF NORTHWESTERN UNIVERSITY

In April 1976 it was recognized that infants delivered at Northwestern Memorial Hospital to substance–abusing women were requiring an inordinate amount of staff time and hospital resources during the time required to recover from the effects of neonatal abstinence. It was at this time that the Perinatal Services Project of Northwestern University was instituted. The purpose of this project was to develop a multidisciplinary, interdepartmental approach to the problems of the addicted pregnant woman and her infant. Although the original concept had been to see only those patients who had been addicted to heroin, and upon admission to the program converted to methadone maintenance, it soon became apparent that services should be expanded to women who were abusers of nonopiate drugs as well. Currently, approximately half the women who present for prenatal addictive and obstetric care are abusers of opiates and half the women use nonopiate substances.

Since mid–1976 close to 200 women and their infants have received care from the Perinatal Services Project. The women enroll in the first or early second trimester of pregnancy and complete a course of intensive prenatal care as described in the previous chapter. Maternal urine samples are obtained regularly to screen for illicit drug use. For neonatal assessment the infants are divided according to the type of primary maternal addiction: heroin/methadone, mixed sedative/stimulant, pentazocine/tripelennamine ('T's and blues'), phencyclidine (PCP) and cocaine.

Women who conceive while on heroin are converted to a variable initial daily dose of methadone upon admission to the program. This dosage is steadily decreased to the lowest level which prevents craving or withdrawal in the mother. By the beginning of the third trimester each woman is on a maintenance dose of methadone which ranges from 5 to 40 mg daily. The average daily dose of methadone in our program is currently 15 mg. The dose is held at a steady level throughout the third trimester of pregnancy, and no woman is completely withdrawn during pregnancy.

Women addicted to multiple licit or illicit nonnarcotic drugs receive the same regimen of prenatal care as opiate-abusing women except that they do not receive methadone maintenance. Women in this group are polydrug abusers in that they tend to use a combination of sedatives and stimulants, including diazepam, marijuana, alcohol and phenobarbital. Although abstinence is the objective for this group, only about 20% of these women remain drug-free throughout the third trimester of pregnancy.

'T's and blues' use became popular in 1979, when heroin was in short supply in the Chicago area. By grinding up tablets of pentazocine (a narcotic) and tripelennamine (a blue antihistamine tablet), putting them into solution and injecting the combination intravenously, it was found that a narcotic-like euphoria could be created. This type of drug use became quite common over a short period of time until heroin was again available. During this period, 15 'T's and blues'-addicted women enrolled in our program for care. All of the women in this group sporadically used other, nonnarcotic drugs, but 'T's and blues' were the only drugs used consistently throughout the pregnancy. Although abstinence was the objective of the program, none of these women remained clean of 'T's and blues' during the third trimester.

Since 1980, 10 women who abused PCP have entered the Perinatal Services Project. All of these women had positive urine screens throughout the first two trimesters of pregnancy, which demonstrated sporadic use of other nonnarcotic drugs in addition to PCP; these were secondary drugs of abuse since use was limited while PCP was used daily by all the women. PCP was the only drug used during the third trimester, and all 10 women had urine screens that were positive for PCP at the time of delivery.

In the past two years there has been an increase in the number of women enrolling in our program who are primary cocaine abusers. These women tend to use alcohol and/or marijuana in addition, and one-third of these women were addicted to heroin at the time of admission to the program. Prenatal management of the women in this group was similar to that for the other groups, including conversion to low-dose methadone maintenance for the heroin-addicted women.

In order to evaluate the effects of drug use on pregnancy and the offspring, 35 women enrolled in the outpatient obstetric clinic of the hospital were recruited to serve as a comparison population for the drug-using women. These women had no history of drug or alcohol abuse, and management of prenatal care and nutrition was similar to that of the drug-abusing women.

All groups of women were evaluated for maternal factors which might affect neonatal outcome: race, maternal age, education, gravidity, prenatal care, nutrition, cigarette smoking and polydrug use. All neonates were examined at birth when weight, length and head circumference were recorded. The BNBAS[27] was administered at 2 – 3 days of age by trained examiners who were blinded to the infants' prenatal history. For long-term follow-up, the Bayley Scales of Infant Development[28] were administered to all infants at 3, 6, 12 and 24 months of age. The infants were examined at these same times, and weight, length and head circumference were recorded. Differences between control and each drug-exposed group of infants at each interval for all parameters of growth and development were then analyzed.

Pregnancy outcome

The incidence of complications usually associated with substance abuse during pregnancy was drastically reduced for all drug-abusing groups of women enrolled in the Perinatal Services program[29]. This was consistent with other studies which have shown that comprehensive care of addicted pregnant women favorably affects pregnancy outcome, especially when methadone maintenance regimes for opiate-addicted women are kept at a daily dose of 20 mg or less.

The only group to exhibit significant problems in pregnancy were those women who used cocaine. The use of cocaine during the first trimester of pregnancy was associated with an increased rate of spontaneous abortions, and third-trimester cocaine use resulted in a high risk of abruptio placentae within 30 minutes of use[30]. The physiologic effects of cocaine that result in tachycardia, vasoconstriction and hypertension are consistent with these third-trimester abruptions, given the recognized association between hypertension and abruptio placentae[31,32].

Fetal growth

Infants delivered to mothers who used narcotics (heroin/methadone, 'T's and blues') had a significantly lower birthweight and length and a smaller head circumference than nondrug-exposed infants[33]. Inasmuch as all the opiate-addicted women in the program were on low-dose methadone maintenance and entered the program early in pregnancy, maternal methadone dosage showed no correlation with fetal growth. The inhibitory effects of heroin on fetal growth[34,35], as well as the effects of inadequate maternal caloric[36] and protein intake[37] can produce fetal growth failure, including effects on brain growth. However, nutritional intake was closely supervised in all women enrolled in the program. It thus appeared that the significant reduction in growth parameters exhibited by the opiate-addicted infants was a direct result of fetal opiate exposure. Intrauterine exposure to nonopiate drugs (sedative/stimulant, PCP, cocaine) apparently did not affect somatic growth parameters of the neonates[30,33].

Neonatal neurobehavior

All infants were evaluated at 2 – 3 days of age with the Brazelton Neonatal Behavioral Assessment Scale (BNBAS), as described above. Infants exposed to drugs *in utero* exhibited significant impairment in their interactive abilities, motor maturity and organizational responses to environmental stimuli (state organization)[30,33]. All the drug-exposed infants were more tremulous and irritable than the control infants, demonstrating significant and unpredictable fluctuations in their emotional reponses. These factors made these infants very difficult to cuddle and comfort, and interrupted the normal processes of maternal/ infant attachment that are so important to the early relationship between infant and mother. PCP-exposed infants were particularly labile and showed marked deficits in their ability to respond to mothering attempts by the caretakers[38].

It is clear from these findings that the behavioral risks that are associated with neonatal narcotic addiction extend to nonopiate-exposed infants as well. These behavioral risks identified at birth with the BNBAS have repercussions for later development inasmuch as infants who have deficits in their ability to maintain a steady state, respond properly to human stimulation and use proper motor control do not respond appropriately to caretaker invitations to interact. Consequently, a vicious cycle of infant passivity and maternal rejection is instituted. It is this cycle which must be interrupted by appropriate intervention if the mother/ infant pair is to successfully interact.

Infant growth

Infants exposed *in utero* to narcotics continued to be significantly smaller in weight and length as compared to the control infants through 6–9 months of age, but by 12 months of age these infants had caught up in weight and length. Head circumference measurements for the opiate-exposed infants did not exhibit such catch-up growth, however, and head circumference for these infants remained significantly smaller than that of the control infants throughout a 2-year follow-up period[33]. The mean head circumference of the nonnarcotic-exposed infants was normal at birth and continued so until 12 months. By 18 months of age, however, head growth of the PCP infants had slowed and fallen to a significantly lower level. The reason for this is unknown but is of concern since small head size in young infants has been reported to be predictive of poor developmental outcome[39] and may be another indicator of the high-risk status of these infants.

Aside from this information, there is very little data regarding longitudinal growth patterns of drug-exposed infants. The nonnarcotic-exposed infants presented here demonstrated normal growth patterns in weight and length throughout the 2-year follow-up period. The narcotic-exposed infants, however, demonstrated early deficits in growth at 3 and 6 months with subsequent catch-up to normals by 12 months of age. This early stunting of growth during the period of subacute withdrawal for the narcotic-exposed infants could be due to the direct effect of methadone on the hypothalamic–hypophyseal axis of the newborn[40]. With the slow excretion of the methadone by the newborn, plasma and tissue drug levels fall, the endocrinological effect of the drug subsides and growth recovers.

Infant development

Two-year developmental follow-up of the drug-exposed infants showed that their development, as measured on the Bayley Scales of Infant Development, was comparable to that of the drug-free infants. Of concern, however, is the fact that all the groups of infants, including the controls, demonstrated a downward trend in developmental scores by 2 years of age[33], a phenomenon not uncommon in infants from a low socioeconomic milieu. From this it appears that the infants' environment and subsequent lack of stimulation had a more direct influence on 2-year development than maternal drug use during pregnancy. More detailed information regarding developmental outcome of these infants is contained in Chapter 9.

Special problems

Infants delivered to women who use drugs during pregnancy remain at risk for various problems beyond the neonatal period. Specific areas of concern include an increased risk of sudden infant death syndrome[41,42], an increased rate of infections[43], and a high rate of child abuse. The problem of increased infections and perhaps a compromised immune system in infants delivered to drug-using women is discussed in Chapter 12, and legal and medical issues related to child abuse are discussed in Chapter 13.

It has been demonstrated that there is a five- to ten-fold increased rate of sudden infant death syndrome (SIDS) among children born to opiate-abusing mothers[41,42]; however, there is no information regarding sudden infant death in populations of infants born to women who use nonnarcotic drugs during pregnancy. Among the first 50 opiate-exposed infants delivered in the Perinatal Services Project, two died of SIDS, a rate (4%) consistent with reports of other authors[41,42]. Due to this high rate of SIDS, a policy was developed by our program in 1982 whereby all infants were to have a screening 24-hour cardiorespiratory recording (pneumogram) made as an outpatient at 8–10 days of age. Each pneumogram is analyzed for all sleep intervals for apnea and periodic breathing using the criteria of Hunt et al.[44]. Any infant with an increased rate of periodic breathing or apnea or periods of prolonged apnea is placed on theophylline therapy at 1.5 mg/kg per dose administered every 6 hours[44], and the pneumogram is repeated. In all cases the pneumogram has converted to normal when a therapeutic level of theophylline has been present. Theophylline therapy is continued until 6 – 8 months of age. The pneumogram is then repeated off medication, and in all cases thus far has reverted to normal. The rate of abnormal pneumograms among the opiate-exposed infants was 4%, similar to the previous rate of SIDS in this population. No infant on theophylline therapy has died of SIDS.

In 1983 it was noted that a sudden increase in the rate of abnormal pneumograms was occurring. An examination of the population enrolled in the program during 1984 and 1985 revealed that among 22 infants delivered to cocaine-using women, 45% had abnormal pneumograms with marked sleep apnea as compared to a rate of 7% among 15 infants delivered to opiate-addicted women during this same period of time. There was no difference between the cocaine- and methadone-exposed infants as to gestational age, birthweight, race or cigarette and alcohol use. It appears that infants delivered to cocaine-using women are at even higher risk for sleep apnea, and perhaps SIDS, than infants delivered to opiate-using women. Although these data are preliminary, they should serve as a warning of cocaine's perhaps fatal effects on the developing fetus and child. No other evidence for an increased rate of SIDS has been documented for other drugs of abuse.

Long-term follow-up

Little reliable information regarding long-term outcomes of infants passively exposed to drugs of abuse is available. To best evaluate these children at school age, environmental factors must be taken into account. These environmental factors are not only socioeconomic but should include aspects of the maternal–infant relationship, including maternal psychopathology and personality. One study which did attempt to control for the caretaking environment of substance-exposed children compared these infants to those whose families began to use drugs after the birth of the children[45]. No differences were found between the *in utero*-exposed children and the children exposed to the social environment of drug-using caretakers. Further studies are needed before final conclusions can be drawn as to the long-term effects of *in utero* drug exposure on infant and child development.

The problems involved in evaluating the effects of the exposure to substances of maternal abuse on the developing fetus and infant are multiple, not the least of which are the difficulties involved in following these infants over a long period of time. The chaotic and transient nature of the drug-seeking environment impairs the early intervention and intensive follow-up necessary to ensure maximum development on the part of each infant. In addition, most women from substance-abusing backgrounds lack a proper model for parenting. These factors, compounded by the early neurobehavioral deficits of the drug-exposed newborns, earmark these infants to be at high risk for developmental and school problems. Maternal and perinatal addiction programs should strive not only to help the mothers deal with their addiction, but to teach them the parenting skills necessary for proper infant stimulation and subsequent development. Future programs must develop methods to ensure adequate follow-up of all infants born to substance-abusing women.

REFERENCES

1. Jones, K. L., Smith, D. W., Ulleland, C. W. and Streissguth, A.P. (1973). Pattern of malformation in offspring of alcoholic mothers. *Lancet*, **1**, 1267 – 71
2. Finnegan, L. P., Connaughton, J. F., Kron, R. E. and Emich, J. P. (1975). Neonatal abstinence syndrome: Assessment and management. In Harbison, R.D. (ed.) *Perinatal Addiction*, pp. 141 – 158. (New York: Spectrum Publications)
3. Chambers, C. D. and Hart, L. G. (1977). Drug use patterns in pregnant women. In Rementeria, J. L. (ed.) *Drug Abuse in Pregnancy and Neonatal Effects*, pp. 73 – 81. (St. Louis: Mosby)
4. Rementeria, J. L. and Nunag, N. (1973). Narcotic withdrawal in pregnancy: stillbirth incidence with a case report. *Am. J. Obstet. Gynecol.*, **116**, 1152 – 6
5. Naeye, R., Blanc, W., Leblanc, W. and Khatamee, M. (1973). Fetal complications of maternal heroin addiction: abnormal growth, infections and episodes of stress. *J. Pediatr.*, **83**, 1055 – 61
6. Connaughton, J. F., Reeser, D., Schut, J. and Finnegan, L. P. (1977). Perinatal addiction: outcome and management. *Am. J. Obstet. Gynecol.*, **129**, 679 – 86
7. Zelson, C. (1973). Infants of the addicted mother. *N. Engl. J. Med.*, **288**, 1393 – 95
8. Reddy, A. M., Harper, R. G. and Stern, G. (1971). Observations on heroin and methadone withdrawal in the newborn. *Pediatrics*, **48**, 353 – 8
9. Zelson, C., Rubio, E. and Wasserman, E. (1971). Neonatal narcotic addiction: 10 year observation. *Pediatrics*, **48**, 178 – 89
10. Desmond, M. M., Schwanecke, R. P., Wilson, G. S., Yasanaga, S. and Burgdorf, I. (1972). Maternal barbiturate utilization and neonatal withdrawal symptomatology. *J. Pediatr.*, **80**, 190 – 7
11. Chasnoff, I. J., Hatcher, R. and Burns, W. J. (1980). Early growth patterns of methadone-addicted infants. *Am. J. Dis. Child.*, **134**, 1049 – 51
12. Chasnoff, I. J. and Burns, W. J. (1984). The Moro reaction: a scoring system for neonatal narcotic withdrawal. *Dev. Med. Child. Neurol.*, **26**, 484 – 9
13. Bleyer, W. A. and Marshall, R. E. (1972). Barbiturate withdrawal syndrome in a passively addicted infant. *J. Am. Med. Assoc.*, **221**, 185 – 6
14. Rementeria, J. L. and Bhatt, K. (1977). Withdrawal symptoms in neonates from intrauterine exposure to diazepam. *J. Pediatr.*, **90**, 123 – 6
15. Athinarayanan, P., Pierog, S. H., Nigan, S. K. and Glass, L. (1976). Chlordiazepoxide withdrawal in the neonate. *Am. J. Obstet. Gynecol.*, **124**, 212 – 13
16. Nichols, M. M. (1967). Acute alcohol withdrawal syndrome in a newborn. *Am. J. Dis. Child.*, **113**, 714 – 15
17. Chasnoff, I. J., Hatcher, R. and Burns, W. J. (1982). Polydrug- and methadone-addicted newborns: a continuum of impairment? *Pediatrics*, **70**, 210 – 13
18. Hill, R. M. and Desmond, M. M. (1963). Management of the narcotic withdrawal syndrome in the neonate. *Pediatr. Clin. N. Am.*, **10**, 67
19. Finnegan, L. P., Connaughton, J. F., Kron, R. E. and Emich, J. P. (1975). Neonatal abstinence syndrome: Assessment and management. *Addict. Dis.*, **2**, 141 – 58
20. Ostrea, E. M., Chavez, C. J. and Stryker, J. C. (1978). *The Care of the Drug Dependent Woman and Her Infant*. (Lansing, MI: Michigan Department of Public Health)
21. Kron, R. E., Litt, M., Phoenix, M. D. and Finnegan, L. P. (1976). Neonatal narcotic abstinence: effects of pharmacotherapeutic agents and maternal drug usage on nutritive sucking behavior. *J. Pediatr.*, **88**, 637 – 41
22. Mitchell, A. A., Louik, C., Lacouture, P., Slone, D., Goldman, P. and Shapiro, S. (1982). Risks to children from computed tomographic scan premedication. *J. Am. Med. Assoc.*, **247**, 2385 – 8
23. Morselli, P. L., Principi, N. and Tognoni, G. (1973). Diazepam elimination in premature and full term infants and children. *J. Perinat. Med.*, **1**, 173 – 6
24. Schiff, D., Chan, G. and Stern, L. (1971). Fixed drug combinations and the displacement of bilirubin from albumin. *Pediatrics*, **48**, 139 – 41

25. Kandall, S. R. (1977). Late complications in passively addicted infants. In Rementeria, J. L. (ed.) *Drug Abuse in Pregnancy and the Neonate*, p. 116, (St. Louis: C. V. Mosby)
26. Finnegan, L.P., Mitros, T. F. and Hopkins, L. E. (1979). Management of neonatal narcotic abstinence utilizing a phenobarbital loading dose method. *Natl. Inst. Drug Abuse Res. Monogr. Ser.*, **27**, 247 – 53
27. Brazelton, T. B. (1976). *Neonatal Behavioral Assessment Scale.* (Philadelphia: Spastics International Medical Publications)
28. Bayley, N. (1969). *Bayley Scales of Infant Development.* (New York: Psychological Corporation)
29. Rosner, M. A., Keith, L. and Chasnoff, I. J. (1982). The Northwestern University Drug Dependence Program: the impact of intensive prenatal care on labor and delivery outcomes. *Am. J. Obstet. Gynecol.*, **144**, 23 – 7
30. Chasnoff, I. J., Burns, W. J., Schnoll, S. H. and Burns, K. A. (1985). Cocaine use in pregnancy. *N. Engl. J. Med.*, **313**, 666 – 9
31. Blair, R. G. (1973). Abruption of the placenta: a review of 189 cases occurring between 1965 and 1969. *J. Obstet. Gynaecol. (Br. Commonw).*, **80**, 242 – 5
32. Pritchard, J. A., Mason, R., Corley, M. and Pritchard, S. (1970). Genesis of severe placental abruption. *Am. J. Obstet. Gynecol.*, **108**, 22 – 7
33. Chasnoff, I. J. (1985). Effects of maternal narcotic vs. nonnarcotic addiction on neonatal neurobehavior and infant development. In Pinkert, T.M. (ed.) *Consequences of Maternal Drug Abuse,* pp. 84 – 95. (Washington, DC: National Institute on Drug Abuse)
34. Taeusch, H. W., Jr., Carson, S. H., Wang, N. S. and Avery, M. E. (1973). Heroin induction of lung maturation and growth retardation in fetal rabbits. *J. Pediatr.*, **82**, 869 – 75
35. Naeye, R. L., Blanc, W. A. and LeBlanc, W. (1973). Heroin and the fetus. *Pediatr. Res.*, **7**, 321
36. Naeye, R. L. and Blanc, W. A. (1973). Maternal nutrition and fetal growth. *Pediatr. Res.*, **7**, 307
37. Winick, M. (1973). Fetal malnutrition and future development. *Pediatr. Ann.*, **2**, No. 4, 10–15
38. Chasnoff, I. J., Burns, W. J., Hatcher, R. P. and Burns, K. A. (1983). Phencyclidine: effects on the fetus and neonate. *Dev. Pharmacol. Ther.*, **6**, 404 – 8
39. Gross, S. J., Oehler, J. M. and Eckerman, C. O. (1973). Head growth and developmental outcome in very low-birth-weight infants. *Pediatrics*, **71**, 70 – 5
40. Friedler, G. and Cochin, J. (1972). Growth retardation in offspring of female rats treated with morphine prior to conception. *Science*, **175**, 654 – 6
41. Pierson, P. S., Howard, P. and Klaber, H. D. (1972). Sudden deaths in infants born to methadone-maintained addicts. *J. Am. Med. Assoc.*, **220**, 1733 – 4
42. Chavez, C. J., Ostrea, E. M., Jr., Stryker, J. C. and Smialek, Z. (1979). Sudden infant death syndrome among infants of drug-dependent mothers. *J. Pediatr.*, **95**, 407 – 9
43. Oleske, J., Minnefor, A., Cooper, R., Thomas, K., de la Cruz, A., Adieh, H., Guerrero, I., Joshi, V. V. and Desposito, F. (1983). Immune deficiency syndrome in children. *J. Am. Med. Assoc.*, **249**, 2345 – 9
44. Hunt, C. E., Brouilette, R. T., Hanson, D., Stein, I. M. and Weissbluth, M. (1985). Home pneumograms in normal infants. *J. Pediatr.*, **106**, 551 – 5
45. Wilson, G. W., McCreary, R., Kean, J. and Baxter, J. D. (1979). The development of preschool children of heroin-addicted mothers: a controlled study. *Pediatrics*, **63**, 135 – 41

6
Marijuana and Human Pregnancy

PETER A. FRIED

There are few plants that lay claim to as interesting and varied a history as marijuana. The wide geographical distribution of this plant is reflected in its many names; in 1968 the United Nations listed 267 terms by which it is known around the world. Kif, dope, hemp, hashish, ganja, dagga, bhang and grass are just a few of its labels. One of the oldest domesticated plants known to man, marijuana has been grown for both utilitarian and intoxicating purposes, dual purposes that have contributed to its fascinating history. The sometimes minor and sometimes major role that marijuana has played in countless societies around the world spans thousands of years and has been described in a most engaging and absorbing manner by Abel[1].

One of the first properties claimed for marijuana in European medicine was its ability to increase contractions during labor and thereby hasten the birth process. Possibly the earliest commissioned scientific report (Marijuana, Indian Hemp Drugs Commission, 1893 – 1984) included in its contents a discussion of marijuana as both a sexual stimulant and, for ascetics, as a sexual inhibitor. The aphrodisiac properties of forms of marijuana are described in sixteenth century Arab literature and also described in the mid-nineteenth century in the *U.S. Dispensatory*, the widely read listing of pharmacological agents of the time. Moving to more recent times, there have been some reports linking marijuana with increased sexual pleasure, but it is not possible to separate the drug's effect from the overall lifestyle of the user and the value placed on sexual activity[2].

There is a fairly large number of scientific reports that have explored the relationship between maternal marijuana ingestion and fetal outcome in a variety of nonhuman species. A critical review of this material has been presented elsewhere[3]. With respect to the human fetus, however, information is comparatively sparse. Constituents of marijuana, including the psychoactive delta-nine-tetrahydrocannabinol (THC), can cross the placenta and be stored in the amniotic fluid[4,5]. That the transfer of these constituents from mother to infant can also take place via the nursing mother is suggested from animal work[6]. This method of potential exposure of the newborn and young infant takes on considerable importance in the human as components of the central nervous system develop extensively postnatally.

THE OTTAWA PRENATAL PROSPECTIVE STUDY

The extreme paucity of information with respect to the effects of marijuana on human pregnancy, the animal work in our own laboratory suggesting *in utero* consequences of marijuana exposure in the developing offspring[7-9], the prevalence of marijuana use by women of reproductive age and the cooperation of a number of hospitals in the Ottawa area led to what has become the Ottawa Prenatal Prospective Study. Since 1978, data have been collected from approximately 700 pregnant women in the Ottawa, Canada, region. Mothers-to-be are informed of the study by their obstetricians and prenatal clinics in the four largest hospitals in the Ottawa region. Upon volunteering to participate and signing an informed consent, each subject is interviewed once during each of the trimesters remaining in her pregnancy. It is important to emphasize the volunteer nature of participation. It is a two-edged sword. This procedure, dictated largely by ethical considerations, limits the generalization of the epidemiological information collected but serves to increase the reliability of the self-report of drug use (elaborated below) and to increase the probability of a long-term commitment to the study. Aside from the subjects who have moved from the Ottawa region (29%), we have maintained a retention rate of over 98% during the past 4 years.

During each of the interviews, conducted in the mother's home in virtually all cases, information is collected concerning sociodemographic status, mother's health (both currently and prior to the pregnancy), father's health history, obstetrical history of previous pregnancies, a detailed listing of all food and drink intake during the 24 hours preceding the interview (including assessment of caffeine intake) and past and present drug use with particular emphasis on marijuana, alcohol and cigarette use. For the establishment of 'soft' drug use, information is gathered both for the year preceding the pregnancy and for each trimester of the pregnancy.

Further details of the interview and the categorization of the various drugs have been described previously[10,11]. Because the range of marijuana use in the sample was quite broad and the drug was not smoked by a uniform number of subjects across the range of usage, the drug data, for descriptive and some statistical purposes, was treated by dividing the subjects into one of four categories[10,12]. There were the nonusers, irregular users (one joint or less per week or regular exposure to the exhaled smoke of others), moderate users (two to five joints per week) and heavy users (more than five joints per week). If the mother-to-be reported using hashish, the number of joints was multiplied by five to take into account the estimated greater concentration of THC in hashish[13].

The demographic details of the participants in the study and the extent of drug use prior to and during pregnancy among the first 407 subjects have recently been published[14], as has a comparison of drug use before, during and after pregnancy[15]. In the present sample 80% of the women stated that they did not use any marijuana in the year before pregnancy, 12% used it irregularly, 3% smoked two to five joints per week and 5% smoked six or more joints per week. Upon becoming pregnant, usage declined significantly, but during each of the trimesters the percentages remained relatively constant with 90% reporting no use, 6% reporting irregular use, 1% smoking two to five joints and 3% reporting six or more joints per week. Compared to alcohol and cigarette use, heavy marijuana consumption was the least reduced during the course of pregnancy. Further, unlike alcohol and cigarette use, which one year after pregnancy was reduced among the heavy users of these drugs compared to prepregnancy levels, heavy marijuana use returned to prepregnancy levels a year after the birth of the baby.

Most of the women who smoked marijuana regularly during pregnancy differed from the remainder of the sample on a number of factors that could be associated with adverse consequences on the course of pregnancy and on the development of the offspring. Among the potential confounding factors were lower socioeconomic level, less formal education and increased cigarette smoking. There was an association between alcohol consumption and heavy marijuana use, but the relationship was not as strong as observed with cigarette smoking. The heavy marijuana users were, on the average, 3.2 years younger than the remainder of the sample; however, no differences in parity were noted. Further, using recommended dietary standards for pregnant women, nutritional adequacy did not differ among the marijuana nonusers and the marijuana users.

COURSE OF PREGNANCY AND PHYSICAL CONGENITAL ANOMALIES

One aspect that we have considered is the effect of marijuana on the course of pregnancy[16]. In our work we found no differences between marijuana users and their matched controls (matched in terms of alcohol use, cigarette use and family income) in terms of rate of miscarriage, type of presentation at birth, Apgar status and the frequency of complications or major physical anomalies at birth. No evidence of increased meconium staining among the newborn of the heavy marijuana users was noted. This is in contrast to the first of two reports by Greenland and his associates[17,18]. In the first of these, the results of an investigation of 35 pregnancies were described. The women included in this investigation reported not using other illicit drugs and were recruited from two California prenatal clinics. Compared to control subjects, a significantly increased incidence of meconium staining among the infants born to marijuana users was found. In their subsequent study the same authors failed to find a similar significant relationship. One of the principal differences in the two studies was a generally higher level of health and

66

living standards among the women who participated in the second study. The sample in the latter report was more similar in terms of ethnicity, education and general health to the Ottawa subjects than were the women in Greenland's first report.

Greenland observed an increased incidence of precipitate labor (less than 3 hours) among the marijuana users in both of his studies (although statistical significance was not obtained in the second investigation). In the Ottawa study a similar trend was noted in that precipitate labor was observed in approximately 25% of the heavy marijuana users as compared to approximately 10% of the nonusers. This possible association between marijuana use and shortened labor is consistent with historical anecdotes described earlier.

The potential importance of the lifestyle of the sample being considered and marijuana's potential effect on pregnancy as suggested by the different findings in Greenland's two reports has support in the animal literature.

Charlebois and Fried[9] exposed rats to either marijuana smoke, placebo smoke or no smoke while manipulating diet. In each of the three drug conditions the animals received one of three diets differing in protein concentration. One diet was relatively poor, one was the standard rat chow and the third was a diet with a higher than usual amount of protein. Both the diet and drug treatments were administered 20 days prior to and throughout gestation. A number of outcomes, including stillbirths, litter destruction and postnatal deaths, were potentiated by a combination of the low-protein diet and marijuana smoke. Interestingly, some physiological and developmental milestones that were delayed in the normal-protein/marijuana smoke condition were attenuated in the high-protein/marijuana smoke condition. It is tempting to speculate, based on this animal work, that marijuana's potential effects may be much more likely to manifest themselves in the human situation in which the lifestyle creates a high-risk environment before the entry of marijuana, and further, in a very low-risk population (of which the Ottawa sample is a case in point), the fetus may be protected from some of marijuana's consequences.

One pregnancy variable that was noted in the Ottawa study was an inverse dose–response relationship between marijuana use and the length of gestation[19]. Use of marijuana an average of six or more times per week during pregnancy was associated with a statistically significant reduction in length of gestation of 1.1 weeks after taking into statistical account nicotine, alcohol, parity, mother's prepregnancy weight and the child's sex. With similar statistical adjustments, no reduction in birthweight was noted once gestational age was taken into account. Once again, this is consistent with the historical description of the medicinal uses mentioned earlier.

The mechanism whereby marijuana may be causing the shortened gestation cannot be specified at this time, although a likely candidate may be the drug's influence upon the reproductive hormonal system. Work with animals has shown that constituents of marijuana can alter a wide

67

range of pituitary–ovarian and adrenal hormones, and possible steroid production by the placenta[3, 20–22].

As mentioned previously, no association between major physical abnormalities and *in utero* marijuana exposure has been found in the Ottawa study. We have also examined the relationship between marijuana and minor physical anomalies[23]. The children of 25 marijuana-using women and the offspring of 25 matched controls were examined for the presence of a large variety of anomalies. None of the anomalies that were looked for occurred significantly more frequently among the offspring of marijuana users, nor were the total number of anomalies present in an individual any higher among the children of marijuana users. Although a pattern of anomalies was not detected among the youngsters born to marijuana users, two anomalies associated with the visual system were found only among the children of the heavy users of the drug. One anomaly was the presence of an unusual amount of skin covering the nasal portion of the eye, and the other anomaly found uniquely among the children born to heavy marijuana users was an unusually wide separation of the eyes.

The lack of a clear relationship between minor physical anomalies and prenatal marijuana exposure is similar to several other recent reports[24,25]. There are, however, two apparent exceptions. One is a large study[26], whereas the second are two reports based on five individual subjects[27,28]. All of these studies examined neonatal outcome in relation to maternal alcohol or marijuana consumption in racially mixed, inner-city samples.

In the reports that found congenital anomalies to be associated with maternal marijuana use, the physical characteristics were those that were part of the diagnostic criteria for the fetal alcohol syndrome[11]. In one report[26] it was stated that the women who smoked marijuana during pregnancy were five times more likely than nonusers to deliver a child with features considered compatible with the fetal alcohol syndrome.

In the case report studies[27,28] a link was also suggested between prenatal marijuana exposure and FAS-type features. In four of the five cases reported, the mothers were regular users of marijuana, but denied use of alcohol or any other psychoactive drugs during pregnancy. The denial of alcohol use by 80% of these subjects is somewhat suspect as virtually all reports in the literature have noted a correlation between regular marijuana use and alcohol consumption[14]. A further difficulty with the case study report is that little demographic or medical history were given and no matching to control potentially confounding factors was undertaken.

The failure to find a significant relationship between FAS features and prenatal marijuana exposure in the Ottawa Prenatal Prospective Study may be due to at least three factors: sample size, age of the subjects and the relative 'risk status' of the women in the study.

First, the sample size in the Ottawa work hindered the finding of significant relationships among the variables studied. This difficulty has been encountered by other researchers in similar studies[17]. In the study in which marijuana offspring were five times more likely than control children to demonstrate features compatible with FAS[26], the rate of occurrence was 2%. If this rate was typical and applied to the Ottawa sample, only one child would be expected to meet the diagnosis.

The subjects in the study linking *in utero* marijuana exposure and FAS features[26] were all examined during the first week after birth. In the Ottawa work, the average age of the subjects was almost 29 months. This difference is an important one as there is considerable evidence that some minor physical anomalies are transient, being seen only during the first few weeks after birth or gradually changing as development proceeds through infancy[29]. The results of European research suggest that features attributed to fetal alcohol exposure may normalize with age, thus suggesting a delay rather than a deficit in development[30].

As described earlier[9], using an animal model, it appears that marijuana use during pregnancy interacts with maternal nutrition to influence fetal outcome. It is therefore consistent that definite physical effects have been reported only in a human sample where poor nutrition (as evidenced by low maternal weight gain during pregnancy) and poor prenatal care are common. The influence of marijuana may be to add to other maternal factors that contribute to putting the fetus at risk. The differences between the Ottawa sample and the sample in which FAS features was noted in the marijuana offspring become crucial. In the latter group of women the maternal weight gain was only 13.64 kg as compared to 16.02 kg among the Ottawa sample. This difference suggests that the Ottawa women were better-nourished than the other sample. Additionally, several other factors combined to place the children of the Ottawa Prenatal Prospective Study at a low risk for environmentally induced congenital anomalies. The mothers lacked any chronic or debilitating diseases, received prenatal care and had a higher socioeconomic status (i.e. 18% of the higher-risk sample had a yearly income of less than $6000 but only 2% of the Ottawa sample did).

INFANT OBSERVATIONS

Published scientific data pertaining to the issue of the possible behavioral effects of *in utero* marijuana exposure are limited to the work arising from the Ottawa Prenatal Prospective Study. The widely used Brazelton Neonatal Behavioral Assessment Scale (BNBAS)[31] is utilized in an effort to quantify the newborn's response to external stimuli, motor organization and ability to regulate alertness. The procedure we followed in the Ottawa Prenatal Prospective Study was to examine the infant at 60–80 hours postpartum, midway between feedings, in a warm, quiet room free from extraneous noises and located close to the hospital nursery.

A number of group differences have been observed using the Brazelton assessment procedure[12,32]. Smoking marijuana regularly during pregnancy was correlated with a marked decrease in the likelihood of the offspring responding to a light repeatedly directed at their eyes. Among the babies born to mothers who had been categorized as heavy users, 46% did not respond to the light, in contrast to 16% of the babies born to matched nonusers. Further, among the offspring of the heavy users that did respond to the light, a third failed to habituate compared to 7% of the matched controls. This was not a general sensorial phenomenon since in a parallel task in the auditory modality, no differences were noted between the marijuana babies and the matched controls.

It is noteworthy that an apparent association between *in utero* marijuana exposure and visual functioning has been reported in previously published primate work[33]. In this work the researchers examined the behavior of the offspring of monkeys who had received daily treatment with THC prior to and during pregnancy and throughout lactation. A variety of behaviors were examined at 1 and 2 years of age. Among them were regulation of activity level, responsiveness to the environment, problem-solving and social interaction. The type of behavior that distinguished the marijuana offspring from the control animals was visual attentiveness. In comparison to the monkeys that had not been exposed to the psychoactive constituent of marijuana, the experimental animals failed to habituate visually to novel visual stimuli. Because only five drug-treated animals were available for observation, the researchers were not able to vary drug dose; nor were they able to separate out whether the effect was a direct effect of prenatal drug exposure on the developing fetal system or an indirect effect mediated by altered maternal physiology and/or behavior. It may also be noteworthy that workers have observed that babies born to methadone-using mothers also responded poorly to visual stimuli but were not abnormal in their responsiveness to auditory stimulation[34,35].

A most consistent and visible consequence of regular heavy marijuana consumption was significantly heightened tremors and startles. Among those offspring born to heavy marijuana users, approximately three-quarters displayed marked tremors (a score of 7 or higher on the Brazelton scale) as contrasted to 30% of matched controls. Startles, both spontaneous ones not elicited by any obvious external stimulation, and elicited ones which arose from experimenter-produced stimuli, were also significantly more pronounced among the babies of the heavy marijuana users.

These state-related findings, together with the altered visual responsiveness, may reflect neurological dysfunction, possibly in the form of nervous system immaturity, or the behavioral observations may be a manifestation of drug withdrawal. However, unlike infants undergoing narcotic withdrawal, the marijuana babies were not more irritable than controls, and they were readily consolable. Finally, at this age, in the Ottawa study no association was noted between the degree of activity or of alertness and maternal marijuana use.

At 9 and 30 days the protocol of the Ottawa study involved the administration of the Prechtl and Beintema neurological examination[36]. By using standardized techniques to elicit a large selection of reflexes and responses, this neurological inventory is designed to measure subtle qualitative and quantitative differences in behavior. The results from this test suggested that the altered visual responsiveness of the visual system observed in the newborn and described above persisted, particularly at 9 days of age, in a significant number of infants born to the heavy marijuana users.

LONG-TERM EFFECTS

As part of the Prechtl examination, various eye movements were also observed, and some abnormalities among the marijuana infants were noted. Because of these observations and the earlier findings involving the visual system of the newborn, a series of neuro-ophthalmological and electrophysiological tests are presently being conducted. Included in this portion of the Ottawa study is a recording of the electrical responses of the visual cortex to a changing checkerboard stimulus and an in-depth examination of the pupillary response, visual tracking ability, acuity and eye movements. Auditory cortical electrical responses are also recorded with the stimuli being various clicks.

The preliminary results are quite suggestive. The dimension of interest in the cortical responses elicited by the visual patterns are the latencies of various components of the waveform. Some parts of the electrical response occur slightly later in children than adults, and the 'mature' waveform appears at about 10 years of age. Among the children born to women who used marijuana during pregnancy, there is a marked tendency for the electrical responses to be slightly slower than control children who are similar in age (3–6 years) and similar with respect to mothers' prenatal use of alcohol and nicotine. This delay is consistent with the notion that prenatal exposure to marijuana may delay the maturation of the visual system. *In utero* exposure to marijuana did not affect the latencies of the cortical responses to auditory stimuli.

The ophthalmological examination has also demonstrated differences among the marijuana subjects and their controls in terms of myopia, strabismus, abnormal eye movements and unusual optic discs. The neuro-ophthalmologist, who examined the children without knowing their prenatal drug exposure history, noted that just over a third of the marijuana subjects had more than one of the above problems as compared to only 6% of the controls.

The Prechtl examinations also revealed state control differences among the babies born to the heavy marijuana users that were consistent with the observations made within the first few days after birth. Most prominent were the marked tremors which, at 9 days of age, were observed in over 40% of the babies contrasted to 12% of the matched controls. At 30 days there were still significant differences, although not as marked as at 9 days. At 1 month marked tremors were noted in 25% of the heavy marijuana offspring as contrasted to approximately 10% of the controls. The tremors among the babies born to the heavy marijuana users were more likely to be low-frequency, high-amplitude in nature, whereas when they did occur in the control babies, they tended to be higher-frequency and lower-amplitude. Some motor differences observed in the offspring of heavy marijuana users included exaggerated reflexes and increased occurrences of writhing movements. Paralleling some of the observations made on the marijuana offspring soon after birth, many of these behaviors were similar to those observed in infants born to women who had used narcotics during pregnancy and whose babies were undergoing withdrawal[35].

In the Ottawa Prenatal Prospective Study the children are administered the Bayley Scales of Infant Development[37] at 6, 12, 18 and 24 months of age. At 18, 24, 36 and 48 months of age the Reynell Expressive Language and Verbal Comprehension Scale[38] is administered, and at 36 and 48 months the McCarthy Scales of Children's Abilities[39] is given.

Group data collected from the tests administered at 6 and 12 months of age failed to differentiate between those babies born to heavy marijuana users and either those born to matched controls or normative scores based on the general population. However, some preliminary findings have been noted. The children born to the heavy marijuana users can be divided into two subgroups. Although the number of subjects that fulfill the criteria for inclusion within the subgroups is small, the results are certainly suggestive. Among those six babies born to heavy marijuana users, and who demonstrated a consistent decrease in visual responsiveness on all three neonatal tests and for whom two Bayley scores are available (at 6 and 12 months), the average score on the mental portion of the Bayley test was 82 (range 60 – 92) at 6 months and 96 (range 75 – 111) at 12 months. Among the seven children who did not show the consistent neonatal decreased visual responsivity, but who were born to mothers with similar heavy marijuana habits, the average score on the mental portion of the 6-month Bayley was 118 (range 106 – 129) and at 12 months was 106 (range 98 – 120). Among matched controls the average scores on these tests was 102 at 6 months and 101 at 12 months. At 18 and 24 months no differences were noted on the mental scores on the Bayley when we compared the offspring of the heavy marijuana users who were consistently visually less responsive as neonates and the children of the heavy marijuana users who had normal visual responses.

An examination of the motor portion of the Bayley test and a breakdown of fine and gross motor tasks at 6, 12, 18 and 24 months failed to reveal any differences between the offspring of the marijuana users and matched controls. Further, subdividing the babies born to mothers who smoked marijuana heavily into those who showed marked tremors on the neonatal tests and those who did not, failed to distinguish the babies on the Bayley motor tests.

CONCLUSIONS

The picture that has emerged to date is that there are a number of neonatal neurobehavioral variables that are correlated with *in utero* marijuana exposure that persist after controlling for nonmarijuana drug habits, the history of previous pregnancies, socioeconomic status and nutritional intake (including caffeine). Further, there are other neonatal symptoms (possibly related to state) that appear to attenuate with age.

Finally, the general observation that the neonatal nervous system alterations seen in the offspring of regular marijuana users does not express itself in a negative fashion on cognitive and motor tests at 1½ and 2 years of age must be interpreted in a conservative fashion. It is not at all clear whether this is the true state of affairs arising because the neurological disturbances present at birth are truly transient and are either overcome or compensated for with maturity, or whether the tests used at these later ages might have a decreased sensitivity to subtle cognitive differences that may actually exist. It may be that the effects of *in utero* marijuana exposure manifest themselves when the child is placed in a situation which places special demands upon nervous system functioning, such as the onset of school. This possibility remains to be investigated.

ACKNOWLEDGEMENT

This work was supported by grants from National Health and Welfare and March of Dimes.

REFERENCES

1. Abel, E. (1980). *Marihuana: The First Twelve Thousand Years*. (New York: Plenum Press)
2. Abel, E. (1981). Marihuana and sex: a critical study. *Drug Alcohol Depend.*, **8**, 1 – 22
3. Fried, P. A. (1984). Prenatal and postnatal consequences of marihuana use during pregnancy. In Yanai, J. (ed.) *Neurobehavioral Teratology*, pp. 275 – 85. (Amsterdam: Elsevier)
4. Harbison, R. and Mantilla-Plata, B. (1972). Prenatal toxicity. Maternal distribution and placenta transfer of tetrahydrocannabinol. *J. Pharmacol. Exp. Ther.*, **180**, 446 – 53.
5. Idanpaan-Heikkila, J., Fritchie, G. E., Englert, L. F., Ho, B. T. and McIsaac, W. M. (1969). Placental transfer of tritiated 1-delta-9-THC. *N. Engl. J. Med.*, **281**, 330
6. Jakubovic, A., Tait, R. M. and McGeer, P. L. (1974). Excretion of THC and its metabolites in ewes milk. *Toxicol. Appl. Pharmacol.*, **28**, 38 – 43
7. Fried, P. A. (1976). Short and long term effects of pre-natal cannabis inhalation upon rat offspring. *Psychopharmacology*, **50**, 185 – 290
8. Fried, P. A. and Charlebois, A. T. (1979). Cannabis administered during pregnancy: First and second generation effects in rats. *Physiol. Psychol.*, **7**, 307 – 10
9. Charlebois, A. T. and Fried, P. A. (1980). The interactive effects of nutrition and cannabis upon rat perinatal development. *Dev. Psychobiol.*, **13**, 591 – 605
10. Fried, P. A., Watkinson, B., Grant, A. and Knights, R. M. (1980). Changing patterns of soft drug use prior to and during pregnancy: A prospective study. *Drug Alcohol Depend.*, **6**, 323 – 43
11. Fried, P. A. (1983). *Pregnancy and Life-Style Habits*. (Toronto: General Publishing)
12. Fried, P. A. (1982). Marihuana use by pregnant women and effects on offspring: an update. *Neurobehav. Toxicol. Teratol.*, **4**, 451 – 4
13. Lerner, M. and Zeffert, J. T. (1968). Determination of tetrahydrocannabinol isomers in marijuana and hashish. *Bull. Narc.*, **20**, 53
14. Fried, P. A., Innes, K. S. and Barnes, M. V. (1984). Soft drug use prior to and during pregnancy: A comparison of samples over a four-year period. *Drug Alcohol Depend.*, **13**, 161–76
15. Fried, P. A., Barnes, M. V. and Drake, E. R. (1985). Soft drug use after pregnancy compared to use before and during pregnancy. *Am. J. Obstet. Gynecol.*, **151**, 787 – 92
16. Fried, P.A., Buckingham, M. and Von Kulmiz, P. (1983). Marihuana use during pregnancy and perinatal risk factors. *Am. J. Obstet. Gynecol.*, **144**, 922 – 4

17. Greenland, S., Staisch, K., Brown, N. and Gross, S. (1982). The effects of marihuana use during pregnancy. I. A preliminary epidemiologic study. *Am. J. Obstet. Gynecol.*, **143**, 408 – 13
18. Greenland, S., Staisch, K., Brown, N. and Gross, S. (1983). Effects of marijuana on human pregnancy, labor, and delivery. *Neurobehav. Toxicol. Teratol.*, **4**, 447 – 50
19. Fried, P. A., Watkinson, B. and Willan, A. (1984). Marihuana use during pregnancy and decreased length of gestation. *Am. J. Obstet. Gynecol.*, **150**, 23 – 7
20. Dalterio, S. and Bartke, A. (1979). Perinatal exposure to cannabinoids alters male reproductive function in mice. *Science*, **205**, 1420 – 2
21. Harclerode, J. (1980). The effect of marihuana on reproduction and development. In Peterson, R. C. (ed.) *Marihuana Research Findings: 1980*, pp. 137 – 66. (Washington: US Govt. Printing Office)
22. Smith, C.G. (1980). Effects of marihuana on neuroendocrine function. In Peterson, R.C. (ed.) *Marihuana Research Findings: 1980*, pp. 120 – 36. (Washington: US Govt. Printing Office)
23. O'Connell, C. M. and Fried, P. A. (1984). An investigation of prenatal Cannabis exposure and minor physical anomalies in a low risk population. *Neurobehav. Toxicol. Teratol.*, **6**, 345 – 50
24. Linn, S., Schoenbaum, S. C., Monson, R. R., Rosner, R., Stubblefield, P. C. and Ryna, K. J. (1983). The association of marijuana use with outcome of pregnancy. *Am. J. Public Health*, **73**, 1161 – 4
25. Rosett, H. L., Weiner, L., Lee, A., Zuckerman, B., Dooling, E. and Oppenheimer, E. (1983). Patterns of alcohol consumption and fetal development. *Obstet. Gynecol.*, **61**, 539 – 46
26. Hingson, R., Alpert, J., Day, N., Dooling, E., Kayne, H., Morelock, S., Oppenheimer, E. and Zuckerman, B. (1982). Effects of maternal drinking and marijuana use on fetal growth and development. *Pediatrics*, **70**, 539 – 46
27. Qazi, Q. H., Mariano, E., Beller, E., Milman, D. and Crumbleholme, W. (1982). Is marijuana smoking fetotoxic? *Pediatr. Res.*, **16**, 272A
28. Qazi, Q. H., Mariano, E., Beller, E., Milman, D., Crumbleholme, W. and Buendia, M. (1983). Abnormalities in offspring associated with prenatal marijuana exposure. *Pediatr. Res.*, **17**, 1534
29. Smith, D. W. (1974). *Recognizable Patterns of Human Malformation*. (Philadelphia: W. B. Saunders)
30. Majewski, F. (1981). Alcohol embryopathy: some facts and speculations about pathogenesis. *Neurobehav. Toxicol. Teratol.*, **3**, 129 – 44
31. Brazelton, T. B. (1973). *Neonatal Behavioral Assessment Scale.* (London: Heinemann)
32. Fried, P. A. (1980). Marihuana use by pregnant women: neurobehavioral effects in neonates. *Drug Alcohol Depend.*, **6**, 415 – 24
33. Golub, M. S., Sassenrath, E. N. and Chapman, C. F. (1981). Regulation of visual attention in offspring of female monkeys treated chronically with delta-9-tetrahydrocannabinol. *Dev. Psychobiol.*, **14**, 507 – 12
34. Lodge, A. (1977). Developmental findings with infants born to mothers on methadone maintenance: a preliminary report. In Beschner, G. and Brotman, R. (eds) *National Institute on Drug Abuse Symposium and Comprehensive Health Care for Addicted Families and Their Children*, pp. 79 – 85. (Washington: US Govt. Printing Office)
35. Finnegan, L.P. (1981). The effects of narcotics and alcohol on pregnancy and the newborn. *Ann. N.Y. Acad. Sci.*, **362**, 136 – 57
36. Prechtl, H. F. R. and Beintema, D. (1969). Neurological examination of the full term infant. *Clin. Devel. Med.*, **12**, 1 – 101
37. Bayley, N. (1969). *Manual for the Bayley Scales of Infant Development.* (New York: Psychological Corporation)
38. Reynell, J. (1969). *Reynell Developmental Language Scale.* (England: Nelson Publishing)
39. McCarthy, D. (1972). *Manual for the McCarthy Scales of Children's Abilities.* (New York: Psychological Corporation)

7
Alcohol Use in Pregnancy

IRA J. CHASNOFF

Although alcohol has long been identified as having a negative effect on pregnancy and the developing fetus, it was not until the American recognition of the syndrome in 1973[1] that widespread acknowledgement of the problem came. Since that time, multiple case reports and studies have confirmed the existence of the fetal alcohol syndrome[2–4]. Unlike other forms of substance abuse in pregnancy, the fetal alcohol syndrome is a clinically observable entity with specific parameters for diagnosis; however, there remain major areas of controversy surrounding the clinical management of the pregnant alcoholic woman and the precise assessment of the impact of alcohol use during pregnancy on the developing fetus and child.

DESCRIPTION OF THE FETAL ALCOHOL SYNDROME

The reported pattern of anomalies in offspring from alcoholic pregnancies is consistent in three particular parameters. These three parameters make up the primary presentation of the fetal alcohol syndrome: (1) prenatal growth deficiency in length and weight, (2) microcephaly, (3) short palpebral fissures.

The range of features attributed to prenatal ethanol exposure is wide. Many of the clinical observations attributed to ethanol teratogenicity, however, have been reported from uncontrolled case studies, and the evidence that they are wholly due to maternal alcoholism is at best circumstantial. Virtually all infants with FAS have very low birthweights for gestational age[5], and body length and head circumference are reduced to a similar degree. Contrary to opiate-exposed infants who are small for gestational age[6], these alcohol-exposed infants do not exhibit catch-up growth and remain small.

The facial similarities of infants and children with FAS are due to a cluster of features associated with midfacial hypoplasia. Short palpebral fissures are easily ascertained by measurement and comparison to data on normal palpebral fissure size for neonates[7]. The reduced size of the palpebral fissures is often due to microophthalmia. Other facial characteristics associated with FAS include epicanthal folds, flat nasal bridge with a short upturned nose, indistinct philtrum, thin vermilion border of the upper lip, hypoplastic maxilla and flattened mid-face. Ptosis and strabismus have also been reported, as well as some malformations of the external ear[1,2,8–11].

Mild to moderate mental retardation is reported frequently, with average IQ scores in several different studies[9,12–17] being around 68, although the range is quite wide. Delayed motor and language development is recognized in early infancy in most cases, and there is no improvement in developmental abilities as the child matures. Hyperactivity, hyperacusis, hypotonia and tremulousness are commonly described in young FAS infants, and symptoms of withdrawal similar to those of narcotic abstinence in neonates have been noted. Evaluation with the Brazelton Neonatal Behavioral Assessment Scale[16,18] reveals that infants born to alcoholic mothers have lower levels of arousal, poor habituation, and are more restless and irritable than control infants.

Disruptions in neonatal state regulation, with a longer latency period before falling asleep and less total time in REM sleep and quiet sleep have also been reported[19,20]. EEG abnormalities consisting of prominent delta bands and atypical slow waves with disorganized background rhythms in the posterior head regions and a significant increase in power in most frequency bands in all stages of sleep have been found in children of heavy drinkers[14,21,22], but the incidence of overt seizures in these children is not increased.

ETIOLOGY OF THE FAS

Since the full FAS is seen in only some of the offspring of chronic alcoholic women, it is reasonable to suspect that a less severe outcome than the full syndrome may arise in other children of overtly alcoholic women and in some infants of moderate drinking women as well. In recent years it has been realized that some infants of frankly alcoholic mothers escape the stigmata of FAS and others have only a few of the characteristics. Those infants with only partial expression are thought to display fetal alcohol effects (FAE)[23]. A simple alcohol dose–response relationship is thus not the answer to the complex issues surrounding the etiology of the FAS.

Animal models have been important in the study of alcohol use in pregnancy, for they provide an opportunity to control for the social variables which plague study designs in humans. Unfortunately, many rodents often cannibalize their abnormal offspring[24], thus impairing evaluation of outcome variables. In addition, extrapolation of animal data to humans is fraught with difficulty in interpreting dosage relationships for small animals in relationship to human dosage. Given these difficulties, animal studies have provided us with some information regarding the effect of alcohol on pregnancy and the fetus.

Several studies in rats have found an increased rate of malformations, an increase in mortality, and a lower birthweight for offspring of alcohol-fed mothers[25-27]. However, not all investigators have reported such positive evidence of ethanol teratogenicity, especially when more moderate doses of alcohol have been used during the prenatal period[28-30]. Neuropathologic studies of the effects of alcohol on fetal rats have revealed evidence of decreased brain weight[31], retarded cerebral cortical lamination[32] and abnormalities of myelination[33], but considerable caution must be exercised in drawing analogies between rodent neuropathic studies and possible similar effects in humans.

Behavioral testing of alcohol-exposed rat pups has resulted in numerous contradictions[34-39], but several studies in animals do correlate with findings of a high incidence of hyperactivity[40] and impaired learning ability[41] similarly reported in human offspring of alcoholic women.

ASSESSMENT OF RISK FOR FAS

In order to assess the risks for the alcoholic woman and evaluate the contribution to this risk of such factors as type, amount, and pattern of alcohol consumption, timing of alcohol use in relation to the pregnancy, and use of cigarettes, marijuana, caffeine and other substances in addition to the alcohol, it is important to realize that FAS represents a spectrum of anomalies that are manifest to a different extent in different individuals. Although several prospective studies have attempted to evaluate a 'safe' level of alcohol use for the pregnant woman, such information is at best speculative, and no clear relationships between quantity of alcohol and severity of infant outcome have been produced. It is likely that the critical aspect is the maximum blood alcohol level attained, and when in pregnancy this occurs. Although the criteria are blurred, the surgeon general of the United States in 1981 recommended that pregnant women abstain from alcohol throughout pregnancy.

Nutrition is a major yet poorly understood factor in the production of the FAS. While the type and adequacy of nutrition varies with socioeconomic and ethnic background, no studies have substantiated the theory that nutritional intake varies in heavy drinkers versus moderate or light drinkers and abstainers when the controls were matched for socioeconomic level and background[42]. However, the efficiency of nutrient utilization is of concern in heavy or light drinkers, since alcoholic impairment of gastrointestinal function has been documented[43].

The association between alcohol use and cigarette smoking has been repeatedly observed[44], and the effects of cigarettes on the developing fetus must be considered in the evaluation of any infant being evaluated for FAS. Smoking women have infants of significantly lower birthweights than nonsmoking women; however, there is no increase in neonatal mortality rate or congenital anomalies among these infants. Of interest, among the many studies relating smoking and low birthweight in these offspring, none took into account that smoking itself was associated with heavier alcohol use; this could have contributed a significant portion of the variance in birthweight.

Use of other drugs, especially marijuana and caffeine, by alcoholic women, is another factor which complicates the evaluation of the effects of alcohol on the fetus. Many commonly used liquid preparations, including cough syrups, mouthwashes and alcohol-based 'tonics', contain appreciable amounts of alcohol and can be associated with changes consistent with FAS[45]. Additionally, alcohol is frequently a secondary drug of abuse. Among the opiate-exposed women enrolled in the Perinatal Addiction Project of Northwestern University, 25% have evidence of concomitant alcohol use.

Differences in fetal susceptibility to ethanol dysmorphogenesis are of prime importance to the expression of the FAS, as has been shown in studies of discordant teratogenesis found in dizygotic twins exposed to similar amounts of alcohol at the same time during gestation[46,47]. The mechanisms underlying this difference in susceptibility could involve discordance of fetal and placental vasculature[48], different rates of organogenesis with resultant differences in susceptibility to teratogenesis at different times[49] or different rates of ethanol degradation and elimination on the part of each fetus[50]. Whatever the mechanism, it is clear that current debates regarding the 'safe' amount of alcohol which can be ingested during pregnancy are futile, since individual fetal susceptibility to dysmorphogenesis is an important yet not predictable factor in the development of the fetal alcohol syndrome. Future research on the teratogenic effects of alcohol should focus on the action of alcohol at the placental and fetal levels rather than only the differences in amounts of alcohol imbibed by the mother.

REFERENCES

1. Jones, K. L., Smith, D. W., Ulleland, C. N. and Streissguth, A. P. (1973). Patterns of malformation in offspring of alcoholic mothers. *Lancet*, **1**, 1267 – 71
2. Hanson, J. W., Jones, K. L. and Smith, D. W. (1976). FAS: Experience with 41 patients. *J. Am. Med. Assoc.*, **235**, 1458 – 60
3. Mulvihill, J. J., Klimas, J. T., Stokes, D. C. and Risemburg, H. M. (1976). Fetal alcohol syndrome: Seven new cases. *Am. J. Obstet. Gynecol.*, **125**, 937 – 41
4. Chernoff, G. F. (1980). A teratologist's view of FAS. *Curr. Alcohol.*, **7**, 7 – 14
5. Streissguth, A. P. Landesman-Dwyer, S., Martin, J. C. and Smith, D. W. (1980). Teratogenic effects of alcohol in humans and laboratory animals. *Science*, **209**, 353 – 61
6. Chasnoff, I. J., Hatcher, R. and Burns, W. J. (1980). Early growth patterns of methadone-addicted infants. *Am. J. Dis. Child.*, **134**, 1049 – 51
7. Fuchs, M., Iosub, S., Bingol, N. and Gromish, D. (1980). Palpebral fissure size revisited. *J. Pediatr.*, **96**, 77 – 8
8. Jones, K. L. and Smith, D. W. (1973). Recognition of fetal alcohol syndrome. *Lancet*, **2**, 999 – 1001
9. Streissguth, A. P., Herman, C. S. and Smith, D. W. (1978). Intelligence, behavior, and dysmorphogenesis in the fetal alcohol syndrome. *J. Pediatr.*, **92**, 363 – 7
10. Oullete, E. M. and Rosett, H. L. (1976). Boston City Hospital study. Part II, the infants. *Ann. N. Y. Acad. Sci.*, **273**, 123 – 9
11. Jones, K. L., Smith, D. W. and Hanson, J. W. (1976). Fetal alcohol syndrome: clinical delineation. *Ann. N. Y. Acad. Sci.*, **273**, 130 – 7

12. Lemoine, P., Haronsseau, H., Borteyru, J. P. and Menuet, J. C. (1968). Les enfants de parents alcoaliques. *Quest. Med.*, **25,** 477 – 82
13. Olegard, R., Sabel, K. G., Aronsson, M., Sandin, B. and Johansson, P. R. (1979). Alcohol abuse during pregnancy. *Acta Paediatr. Scand. (Suppl).*, **275,** 112 – 21
14. Root, A. W., Reiter, E. O., Andriola, M. and Duckett, G. (1975). Hypothalamic and pituitary function in the fetal alcohol syndrome. *J. Pediatr.*, **87,** 585 – 8
15. Streissguth, A. P., Herman, C. S. and Smith, D. W. (1978). Stability of intelligence in FAS. *Alc. Clin. Exp. Res.*, **2,** 165 – 70
16. Streissguth, A. P., Landesman-Dwyer, S., Martin, J. C. and Smith, D. W. (1980). Teratogenic effects of alcohol in humans and laboratory animals. *Science*, **209,** 353 – 61
17. Jones, K. L., Smith, D. W., Streissguth, A. P. and Myrianthopoulos, N. C. (1974). Outcome in offspring of chronic alcoholic mothers. *Lancet*, **1,** 1076 – 8
18. Landesman-Dwyer, S., Keller, L. S. and Streissguth, A. P. (1978). Naturalistic observations of newborns: effect of maternal alcohol consumption. *Alc. Clin. Exp. Res,* **2,** 171 – 7
19. Sander, L. W., Snyder, P. A. and Rosett, H. L. (1977). Effects of alcohol intake during pregnancy on newborn state regulation. *Alc. Clin. Exp. Res.*, **1,** 233 – 41
20. Rosett, H. L., Snyder, P., Sander, L. W., Lee, A., Cook, P. and Weiner, L. (1979). Effects of maternal drinking on neonate state regulation. *Dev. Med. Child Neurol.*, **21,** 464 – 73
21. Havlicek, V. and Childeava, R. (1976). Letter. *Lancet*, **2,** 477
22. Havlicek, V., Childeava, R. and Chernick, V. (1977). EEG frequency spectral characteristics of sleep states in infants of alcoholic mothers. *Neuropaediatrie,,* **8,** 360 – 73
23. Clarren, S. K. and Smith, D. W. (1978). The fetal alcohol syndrome. *N. Engl. J. Med.*, **298,** 1063 – 7
24. Buckalew, L. W. (1978). Problems in the use of rodents for studies of maternal exposure to ethanol. *Psychol. Rep.*, **43,** 1313 – 14
25. Kronick, J. B. (1976). Teratogenic effects of ethyl alcohol administered to pregnant mice. *Am. J. Obstet. Gynecol.*, **124,** 676 – 80
26. Randall, C. L. and Taylor, W. J. (1979). Teratogenic effects of prenatal ethanol exposure in mice. *Teratology*, **19,** 305 – 12
27. Sherwin, B. T., Jacobson, S., Troxell, S., Rogers, A. and Pelham, R. (1980). Rat model of FAS. *Curr. Alcohol.*, **7,** 15 – 30
28. Schwetz, B. A., Leong, B. T. and Staples, R. E. (1975). Abstract. *Teratology*, **11,** 33A
29. Schwetz, B. A., Smith, F. A. and Staples, R. E. (1978). Teratogenic potential of ethanol in mice, rats and rabbits. *Teratology*, **18,** 385 – 92
30. Oisund, J. F., Fjorden, A. E. and Morland, I. (1978). Is moderate ethanol consumption teratogenic in the rat? *Acta Pharmacol. Toxicol.*, **2,** 145 – 55
31. Anderson, W. J. (1979). Alcohol induced defects in cerebeller development in the rat. *Alc. Clin. Exp. Res.*, **2,** 192
32. Jacobson, S., Rich, J. and Tousky, N. (1979). Delayed myelination and lamination in cortex of rats due to fetal alcohol syndrome. *Curr. Alcohol.*, **5,** 123 – 33
33. Dryse, M. J. and Hoftieg, J. H. (1977). Maternal alcohol consumption and development of CNS myelination subfractions in rats. *Drug Alc. Depend.*, **2,** 421 – 9
34. Abel, E. L. (1975). Emotionality in offspring of rats fed alcohol while nursing. *J. Stud. Alcohol*, **36,** 654 – 8
35. Yanai, J. and Ginsburg, B. (1976). Audiogenic seizures in mice whose parents drank alcohol. *J. Stud. Alcohol*, **37,** 1564 – 71
36. Yanai, J. and Ginsburg, B. (1979). Contributions of pre- and post-natal ethanol administration to changes in mice behavior. *Arch. Int. Pharmacodyn.*, **241,** 235 – 44
37. Branchly, L. and Friedhoff, A. J. (1976). Biochemical and behavior changes in rats exposed to ethanol in utero. *Ann. N. Y. Acad. Sci.*, **273,** 328 – 30
38. Ewart, F. G. and Cutler, M. G. (1979). Effects of ethyl alcohol on development and social behavior in the offspring of laboratory rats. *Psychopharmacologia*, **62,** 247 – 51
39. Riley, E. P., Shapiro, N. R. and Lochry, E. A. (1979). Nose-poking and head-dipping behavior in rats prenatally exposed to ethanol. *Pharmacol. Biochem. Behav.*, **11,** 513 – 9
40. Brose, D. H. and Loh, H. H. (1975). 5-hydroxytryptamine and minimal brain dysfunction. *Life Sci.*, **16,** 1005 – 16

41. Shaywitz, B. A., Klopper, J. H. and Gordon, J. W. (1976). Syndrome resembling minimal brain dysfunction in rat pups of alcoholic mothers. *Pediatr. Res.,* **10,** 450

42. Kaminski, M., Rumeau-Rouquette, C. and Schwartz, D. (1976). Alcohol consumption among pregnant women and outcome of pregnancy. *Rev. Epidemiol. Sante Publique,* **24,** 27 – 40

43. Moghissi, K. S. (1978). Maternal nutrition in pregnancy. *Clin. Obstet. Gynecol.,* **21,** 297 – 310

44. Streissguth, A. P., Barr, H. M. and Martin, D. C. (1980). The effects of maternal alcohol, nicotine, and caffeine use. *Alc. Clin. Exp. Res.,* **4,** 152

45. Chasnoff, I. J., Diggs, G. and Schnoll, S. H. (1981). Fetal alcohol effects and maternal cough syrup abuse. *Am. J. Dis. Child.,* **135,** 968

46. Christoffel, K. K. and Salafsky, I. (1975). Fetal alcohol syndrome in dizygotic twins. *J. Pediatr.,* **87,** 963 – 7

47. Chasnoff, I. J. (1986). Fetal alcohol syndrome in twin pregnancy. *Acta Genet. Med. Gemellol.* **34,** 229 – 32

48. Fogel, B. J., Nitkowsky, H. M. and Gruenwald, P. (1965). Discordant abnormalities in monozygotic twins. *J. Pediatr.,* **66,** 64 – 72

49. Lenz, W. (1966). Malformations caused by drugs in pregnancy. *Am. J. Dis. Child.,* **112,** 99 – 105

50. Seppala, M., Raiha, N. C. R. and Tamminen, V. (1971). Ethanol elimination in a mother and her premature twins. *Lancet,* **1,** 1188 – 9

8
Psychotropic Drugs in Pregnancy

LAWRENCE L. KERNS and GILLA P. DAVIS

Pregnancy is frequently complicated by the development or recurrence of a serious mental disorder; neurotic, major affective, and psychotic illnesses have all been observed[1-4]. When a major mental disorder arises in a pregnant woman and threatens her life, health, or that of the fetus, it should be treated early and aggressively to minimize complications and forestall the advance of the disease. Nonbiologic methods like individual psychotherapy, couples or family therapy, social casework, and hospitalization in a supportive, structured milieu should form the first line of treatment. If the illness persists in spite of nonbiological interventions, and if the risks of the inadequately treated disease outweigh the risks associated with a potentially useful medication, then a trial of that medication is clearly indicated.

However, the physician's dilemma occurs because although as many as 80% of pregnant women take prescribed drugs, and up to 35% take a psychoactive drug[5,6], no psychotropic drug has been proven safe for use during pregnancy, and all carry warnings by the FDA[7]. Furthermore, in calculating the medication's risks, the physician must rely mostly on animal data and suboptimal human epidemiologic studies. In this chapter we will first review the types of risk posed to mother and fetus by drugs in general, with special attention to the features of maternal and fetal physiology which increase those risks. We will then consider the risks and benefits associated with antipsychotics, antidepressants, and lithium, suggesting guidelines for their use in the pregnant patient.

Maternal physiology and risk

For those patients requiring drug treatment, the risks to the mother are similar to the risks posed to the nonpregnant patient, but compounded by the metabolic, endocrine, renal and cardiac changes in pregnancy. Delayed gastric emptying and increased intestinal transit time may lead to slower but more complete drug absorption. Plasma volume, total body water and body fat are increased, resulting in a higher volume of distribution and a lower serum concentration for any given dose of drug. This increases the volume of fluid which the kidney must in some cases clear of drug[8]. This may or may not be counterbalanced by the steady increase in renal blood flow and glomerular filtration rate which tend to speed the clearance of free drug. Although albumin production is normal or increased, plasma albumin concentration falls and total plasma drug concentration is decreased. If the total circulating albumin is reduced, as by pre-eclampsia or the nephrotic syndrome, binding sites can become saturated and free drug fraction rises[9]. The hormonal milieu of pregnancy is thought to increase metabolic activity in the liver[8] and may tend to speed breakdown of some drugs.

Fetal physiology and risk

Further complicating the use of drugs in pregnancy is the presence of an additional but equally complex patient, the fetus. All psychotropic drug classes cross the placenta. Transfer occurs primarily by simple diffusion, dependent upon the chemical properties of the drug (including molecular size, protein-binding affinity, polarity and lipid solubility), drug concentration and duration of exposure[10]. Non-ionized, low molecular weight, lipid-soluble drugs are well absorbed. Placental metabolism of drugs is probably less active than metabolism within the fetal liver. Intended or unintended drug effects may act to reduce placental blood flow or interfere with active transport and other nutritive functions of the placenta.

Compared to the adult, fetal cardiac output is greater and a higher proportion of blood flow is distributed to the brain. Combined with greater blood–brain permeability this leads to more rapid and more complete drug exposure of the fetal brain[11]. Total concentration of plasma protein and protein-binding affinity are less in the fetus than in the mother, leaving more free drug available for tissue penetration and competition with other drugs and endogenous compounds for protein binding[10]. Drugs are metabolized chiefly in the fetal liver, where the activity and concentration of certain microsomal enzymes is less than in the adult, prolonging and exaggerating drug effects. Excretion of most drugs, via the placenta and fetal urine, is delayed.

Like the fetus, the neonate has proportionally less total serum protein for binding, less active hepatic degradative enzymes, and a lower glomerular filtration rate than the adult. The blood–brain barrier is still incomplete and the immature CNS appears generally more sensitive to drug effects[10]. Furthermore, the neonate no longer exists in equilibrium with its mother via the placenta, and a drug concentrated in the fetus shortly before birth may have significantly prolonged postnatal effects.

The risks to the fetus include teratogenic effects, long-term neurobehavioral effects and direct toxic effects. A teratogenic effect may be immediate or delayed; it may consist of abortion, malformation, altered fetal growth, functional deficit, carcinogenesis or mutagenesis. Psychotropic drugs can also produce long-term functional effects which are not accompanied by gross structural malformations and which may not be measurable or manifest for years after birth. Since the pioneering studies of Werboff and colleagues established the field of behavioral teratology,[12,13] numerous subsequent animal studies have shown that prenatal exposure to a variety of psychoactive drugs can disturb nerve cell proliferation and differentiation[14], neurotransmitter concentrations[15], and behavioral development and performance[16,17]. Such psychoteratogenicity may be expressed as disturbed psychomotor activity, faulty adaptation to the extrauterine environment, abnormal learning or problem-solving capacity, or other subtle cognitive deficits and mood disturbances.

However, attention has been given to studying the long-term neuro-behavioral and psychological effects in humans of prenatal exposure to the antipsychotics, antidepressants and lithium. The few follow-up studies available will be discussed under the drug classes to which they apply, but the clinician should be aware that our knowledge in this area is inadequate, and the implications for exposed offspring are potentially grave. Not only is caution in prescribing advised, but long-term, systematic follow-up of the children is crucial.

To date all human studies on the effects of psychotropic drugs in pregnancy suffer from poor control of potentially confounding variables such as maternal age, gravidity and parity as well as history of miscarriages, stillbirths and prior malformed infants. Maternal nutrition, alcohol use, cigarette use and over-the-counter and prescription drug use all need to be carefully controlled or at least matched. The dose of drug, duration of exposure and timing of exposure are critical variables, exemplified by thalidomide's ability to produce limb defects only between the 42nd and 48th days of gestation[18]. Thus a study which combines all first-trimester drug exposures may miss a subtle effect produced only during a brief gestational 'window.' The mother's illness and the indication for drug use is another often-neglected variable. Many of the studies on phenothiazine effects were carried out on patients with nausea and vomiting rather than a mental disorder. Not only are the doses low and brief, but as psychiatrists we have no comparison of the morbidity and mortality of treated versus untreated maternal mental illness. Finally, the length and depth of follow-up is generally inadequate. As Edlund and Craig[19] have shown, the cumulative incidence of congenital anomalies increases with increasing length of follow-up. Therefore if we hope to detect subtle or delayed neurobehavioral effects in children exposed prenatally to psychotropic drugs, our observations must be both thorough, in terms of neurobehavioral assessment techniques, and extended, ideally into adulthood.

ANTIPSYCHOTIC DRUGS

Indications

The antipsychotic drugs have repeatedly been shown effective in the treatment of acute psychotic episodes occurring in schizophrenic, affective, and a variety of other mental disorders. They have been used effectively to treat psychotic symptoms in pregnant women as well. Such symptoms as hallucinations, delusions or profound disorientation respond well to antipsychotics.

Adverse effects on mother

Sedation, postural hypotension, anticholinergic and extrapyramidal symptoms may occur. Anticholinergic effects on the bowel may worsen the constipation which is common in pregnancy. Likewise the sedative effect may compound the pregnant woman's fatigue. Most important, however, is the potential effect on maternal blood pressure, and the potential compromise of placental blood flow should always be kept in mind. The risk of tardive dyskinesia of course always pertains.

Teratogenic effects

Phenothiazines and thiozanthenes have been shown to pass the placental barrier, and phenothiazines have been measured in various concentrations in fetal brain and liver.

Most reviews of the use of chlorpromazine, haloperidol or perphenazine in human pregnancy find no statistically significant increase in the incidence of major congenital structural malformations in exposed offspring[20-27]. In a prospective survey of 12 764 pregnant women, Rumeau-Rouquette and associates[28] found a statistically significant increase in the number of infants born with major malformations when exposed prenatally to phenothiazines with a 3-carbon aliphatic side-chain (chlorpromazine, methotrimeprazine, trimeprazine and oxomemazine). Compared to non-exposed controls, a similar increase was not observed with promethazine or the piperazine and piperidine antipsychotics. Of the implicated drugs, only chlorpromazine is used as an antipsychotic in the United States, and although this study might provide reason for avoiding chlorpromazine, many confounding factors among those women were not considered. Probably the best controlled study to date is the one by Milkovich and Van den Berg[29]. Among 20 504 pregnant women followed prospectively, 19 952 were treated for nausea and vomiting during their first trimester, mostly with phenothiazines and especially prochlorperazine. Maternal age, type of drug and gestational age at exposure were controlled. They found no increase in the rates of severe congenital anomaly and perinatal death for the exposed group compared to controls. However, no doses were recorded and compliance was not assessed. When used as antiemetics the phenothiazines are likely to be used intermittently and in lower doses than those needed for the treatment of psychosis.

Long-term neurobehavioral effects

Animal studies have found that prenatal exposure to antipsychotic drugs can affect vasculogenesis[30-36], neurogenesis[37,38], central catecholamine levels[15], and dopamine receptor function[33]. Some animal studies report persistent abnormalities of learning behavior[16,34,35], while others do not[36]. Data on long-term behavioral consequences in humans are scarce.

After several case reports of persistent neurobehavioral abnormalities in infants of mothers treated with phenothiazines[37], Desmond and associates[38] reported on 19 infants born to mothers on phenothiazines. Agitation and hypertonicity persisted for several months after birth. Many of these infants were also exposed to alcohol and barbiturates *in utero*, however, and the effect could not be attributed to a single drug. Stone *et al.*[27] found no difference in IQ scores at 4 years of age between 151 children exposed to phenothiazines *in utero* and controls who were not exposed. Kris[39] followed 52 children exposed to low doses (50–150 mg/day) of chlorpromazine prenatally, and found no behavioral or intellectual abnormalities. However, these represent small samples of children, generally exposed to low doses of antipsychotic medication at variable times in gestation, and better-controlled, more rigorous follow-up studies are needed.

Direct toxic effects on the fetus and neonate

Direct toxic effects of antipsychotic drugs which have been observed in newborns include motor restlessness, abnormal movements, hypertonia, and tremor[37,40–42]. Functional bowel obstruction and neonatal jaundice have also been described[43]. *In vitro* studies have raised the possibility of toxic effects on chromosomes[44], lymphocytes[45], and the fetal retina[46].

Recommendations

For the women with a chronic psychotic disorder or at risk for an acute psychotic episode during pregnancy, early comprehensive obstetrical and psychiatric management and social support should be instituted. Crisis intervention techniques are useful at the first sign of deterioration. If the patient is unstable, hospitalization and use of a therapeutic milieu should be tried first.

If psychotic symptoms severe enough to threaten the life or health of the woman or her fetus persist in spite of aggressive nonbiologic treatment, the use of an antipsychotic drug is indicated, but delay is recommended through the first trimester if at all possible. Obtain informed consent from the patient and her spouse if feasible. In choosing a drug, consider the patient's prior drug response and tolerance of side-effects, or that of family members if applicable. Use the side-effect profile of the antipsychotic drug to optimize treatment of the patient's symptoms. If she is profoundly agitated and sleepless, choose a low-potency drug like thioridazine or chlorpromazine, but beware of hypotensive effects. Otherwise, a high-potency agent like haloperidol or fluphenazine is generally preferred. Give a low initial test dose and increase cautiously until the minimum effective dose is reached.

The treatment goal is sufficient control of symptoms to ensure the safety of the woman and her fetus to term; it is not necessary or advisable to strive for complete eradication of symptoms. Anticholinergic medications may be used if necessary for treatment of extrapyramidal symptoms, but these have potential for toxic effects on the fetus. Avoid the use of other medications.

There is considerable evidence that maintenance use of antipsychotic medications after remission of the acute phase helps prevent relapse, but maintenance drug treatment should be based on the severity of symptoms, the chronicity of the illness, and availability of social support systems. Consider the natural history of the individual patient's illness, and reduce or discontinue the medication if at all possible.

ANTIDEPRESSANTS

Indications

Heterocyclic antidepressants are generally the treatment of first choice for major depression and the depressed phase of bipolar disorder. They have also found therapeutic usefulness in dysthymic disorders, atypical depressions, personality disorders with depressed mood, panic and phobic disorders, obsessive–compulsive disorders, chronic pain syndromes, and depression in schizophrenia and schizo-affective disorders. They may be indicated in pregnancy when the mother's depression is severe enough to threaten the life and health of herself and her fetus. This includes suicidal intent, vegetative and nutritional disturbance, or severely impaired functioning and judgement not responsive to nonbiological interventions including hospitalization.

Adverse effects on the mother

These include anticholinergic effects (dry mouth, decreased GI motility, mydriasis, cycloplegia, urinary hesitancy or retention, tachycardia and, in high doses, delirium), orthostatic hypotension and sedation. Imipramine and other tertiary amines more commonly cause hypotension and should generally be avoided in favor of less hypotensive drugs.

Teratogenic effects

Imipramine and desipramine have been shown to cross the placenta in animals and humans. In at least one animal study imipramine and desipramine were found to cross the placenta and to potentiate the pressor response to norepinephrine while amitriptyline and protriptyline did not. Van Petten[47] noted that even closely related compounds can show differences in penetration of the placenta and subsequent pharmacologic effects on the fetus. Demonstration of such differences in human pregnancies in the future could facilitate the choice of the antidepressant safest for the fetus.

Sporadic case reports suggesting a possible association between maternal imipramine or amitriptyline use and fetal limb reduction deformities have appeared in the literature[48,49]. One retrospective case control study of 2784 cases of birth defects was inconclusive[50], while other small cohort[51–54] studies found no causal relationship between maternal imipramine or amitriptyline intake and congenital anomalies in the offspring.

Long-term neurobehavioral effects

Animal studies have clearly demonstrated that prenatal exposure to tricyclic antidepressants, in therapeutic doses, can produce behavioral and neurochemical disturbances lasting well past termination of drug exposure and into adulthood. Rats exposed prenatally to imipramine show decreased hypothalamic dopamine levels and decreased cortical beta-adrenergic receptors[55], delayed reflex development and decreased exploratory responses[56], and reduced physiological and behavioral responsiveness as adults[57]. Similar results have been obtained after prenatal clomipramine exposure[58]. Early neonatal treatment of rats with a monoamine oxidase inhibitor has resulted in nerve cell changes and decreased concentrations of norepinephrine and dopamine in the hypothalamus, reduced learning capacity, and diminished emotional reactivity in later life[59 – 61].

Neurobehavioral follow-up studies in humans have not been done.

Recommendations

Antidepressants should be reserved for the pregnant woman whose depression is severe enough to threaten the life and health of herself and her fetus, and which is unresponsive to nonbiologic interventions. Reactive depressions or biological depressions that are less severe should be treated with psychotherapy alone or in a therapeutic milieu. A careful history, especially of cardiac diseases, review of systems, physical exam and EKG should precede the initiation of treatment. Inquire about a prior response to a specific antidepressant.

In general, avoid the tertiary amines (imipramine, amitriptyline) because of their increased hypotensive effects. A reasonable choice for cardiac safety is trazodone if sedation is desired, desipramine if it is not. These drugs have relatively low anticholinergic effects as well. Begin with a low dose and increase slowly, using plasma drug levels and clinical response to achieve the minimal dose effective in relieving the major depressive symptoms. Monitor pulse, orthostatic blood pressure changes, and EKG if any abnormality is found on the baseline EKG. Give the entire daily dose at bedtime if daytime sedation is to be avoided or nighttime sedation desired. Divide or reduce the dose if the patient develops hypotension, hypertension, arrhythmias, fainting, or heart failure. Persistent adverse cardiovascular effects may necessitate stopping the drug.

Avoid co-administration of other drugs, over-the-counter or prescription, especially those that affect the cardiovascular system. If at all possible, avoid the use of antidepressants during the first trimester, and attempt to reduce or discontinue the medication before term. There is a particularly high risk of depression in the postpartum period, when resumption of medication and avoidance of breastfeeding may be indicated.

LITHIUM

Indications

Lithium is the drug of choice for prophylaxis against bipolar affective episodes of the manic type. It also carries FDA approval for use in acute manic episodes and in prophylaxis against the depressive phase of bipolar disorder. It may also be useful in acute depression for patients who are unresponsive to other somatic treatments, as prophylaxis against recurrence of schizo-affective illness, in disorders of impulse control and episodic violence, and possibly in some alcoholics.

Approximately one-half of patients with bipolar disorder are women, and the first manic episode typically occurs before age 30, well within the limits of a woman's reproductive life. Women may first manifest the disorder during a pregnancy, and may have up to 50% risk of developing a postpartum psychosis which can appear from days to weeks following the birth[2]. Practitioners in obstetrics and in general psychiatry will undoubtedly encounter pregnant patients with bipolar disorder.

Adverse effects on mother

Lithium presents the same spectrum of side-effects and adverse reactions for pregnant women as for others (endocrine, renal, gastrointestinal, neurologic), but physiological changes in pregnancy may increase the relative risk. Progressively increasing lithium clearance by the kidney may require increasing lithium doses to maintain a desired serum concentration. The precipitous fall in glomerular filtration rate and lithium clearance after delivery may leave the patient toxic[62]. The use of thiazide diuretics or sodium restriction to treat hypertension or edema of pregnancy may change the fluid and electrolyte balance and quickly lead to maternal and fetal lithium toxicity[63].

Teratogenic effects

Lithium freely crosses the placenta, and the concentration in cord blood equals that of maternal serum.

Lithium has repeatedly been shown to be teratogenic in premammalian species, causing abnormal tissue differentiation, disorganized CNS development, and head and neck anomalies[64]. Studies in non-human mammals are contradictory, one showing lithium to be teratogenic[65] while others do not[64]. One study showed an adverse effect on human chromosomes *in vitro* but lithium levels used were in the toxic range.

In order to assess the possible teratogenic effect of lithium in humans, the International Register of Lithium Babies was begun in 1968. Although the incidence of malformations in babies of untreated mothers with affective disorders is unknown, and although a study of this design cannot produce a true incidence of malformations, pathologic trends may be revealed[66]. Consecutive reports from 1971 to 1975 revealed increasing likelihood that lithium exerts a teratogenic effect in humans, especially on the developing cardiovascular system[67-69]. As of 1980, 225 babies exposed to lithium in the first trimester of pregnancy had been reported to the register, 25 of whom were born with congenital malformations. Besides one baby with intracerebral toxoplasmosis, two with Down's syndrome, and seven stillborn, 18 of the 25 babies with congenital malformations had involvement of the heart and great vessels, six of them the exceedingly rare Ebstein's anomaly (comprising defects of the tricuspid valve, atrial septum, and right ventricle). Lithium, when administered in the first trimester, is therefore felt likely to be teratogenic with respect to the cardiovascular system.

Long-term neurobehavioral effects

A study of behavioral effects on rats exposed to lithium *in utero* showed a significant decrease in performance on a T-maze and changes in avoidance behavior[70], but animal studies may not reflect the effects on humans. A case report exists of developmental motor delay persisting at 1 year of age in a human infant found to be lithium toxic at birth, but it is not clear whether the motor delay was due to high lithium levels at birth or due to cerebral hypoxia associated with lithium-induced cardiac hypofunction[71]. A follow-up of 60 lithium children not malformed at birth did not reveal any significantly increased frequency of physical or mental anomalies in the lithium children as compared to sibling controls[72] but conclusions were based only on mothers' subjective assessments, not actual examination or neurobehavioral testing.

Direct toxic effects on the fetus and neonate

Several authors have reported neonatal toxicity in the offspring of mothers on toxic or even therapeutic doses of lithium at the time of delivery[63,73,74]. Findings in the neonate include: cyanosis, muscle flaccidity and hypotonia, poor suck and grasp reflexes, absent Moro reflex, and lethargy which may take up to 10 days to resolve. Other adverse effects reported in the neonate include atrial flutter[75], functional tricuspid regurgitation and congestive heart failure[76], reversible inhibition of fetal thyroid[77], and nephrogenic diabetes insipidus which persisted for 2 months after birth[78].

Recommendations

Lithium should be used in pregant women only for unequivocal indications, and only after careful consideration of all potential risks and benefits. Women with a history of bipolar disorder have a high risk of developing a manic episode off lithium, as studies have shown that 70% of patients will have at least one relapse within a year of discontinuing lithium versus 20% of those who are maintained on lithium. A pregnant woman in an acute manic phase can do serious harm to herself and her fetus. On the other hand, use of lithium carries multiple potential serious risks to both mother and child as outlined above.

Women on lithium should be urged to avoid pregnancy and to maintain effective contraception. One who plans to become pregnant or who inadvertently becomes pregnant should be withdrawn from lithium prophylaxis during the first trimester unless there is convincing evidence that doing so would endanger the woman or her fetus. The decision to institute, continue, or discontinue lithium administration in a woman for whom pregnancy is a fact or a possibility should be made with the collaboration and informed participation of both the patient and her husband.

If a pregnant woman develops an acute manic episode, hospitalization with a structured, supportive milieu and regular individual psychotherapy would be indicated first. Judging by currently available evidence, antipsychotic drugs are probably safer than lithium in the first trimester, and more rapidly effective for acute manic symptoms. Choose a low-dose, high-potency agent at the lowest dose effective in alleviating dangerous symptoms.

If it is believed safest for the woman and her fetus to institute lithium treatment after the first third or half of pregnancy, use the minimum dose necessary to achieve the desired therapeutic or prophylactic effect, achieving a serum level of 0.7 – 1.2 mg Eq/l in most cases. A single lithium dose should not exceed 300 mg, given as often as necessary to achieve the target serum concentration. This avoids 'pulses' of lithium which may be more harmful to the fetus than a steady serum concentration. Serum lithium levels should be closely monitored, as often as weekly towards the end of pregnancy and even more frequently in the days before term. Monitor thyroid status during pregnancy and use thyroid supplement as needed to protect mother and fetus against goiter formation. Sodium-depleting diuretics should not be used; sodium-restricted diets should be used only with great caution. Reduce the daily lithium dose by 50% in the last week of gestation and stop completely at the onset of labor. Reinstitute lithium at prepregnancy dosage (or 50% of the term dosage if no prepregnancy dose was established) as soon after delivery as fluid homoeostasis is re-established, usually 3 days.

REFERENCES

1. Kumar, R. and Robson, K. (1978). Neurotic disturbance during pregnancy and the puerperium: preliminary report of a prospective survey of 119 primiparae. In: Sandler M. (ed.) *Mental Illness in Pregnancy and the Puerperium*. (Oxford: Oxford University Press)
2. Targum, S. D. (1979). Dealing with psychosis during pregnancy. *Am. Pharmacol.*, **N.S. 19,** 18 – 21
3. Molinski, H. A.: Masked depressions in obstetrics and gynecology. *Psychother. Psychosom.* **31,** 283 – 7
4. Cox, J. (1979). Psychiatric morbidity and pregnancy: a controlled study of 263 semi-rural Ugandan women. *Br. J. Psychiatry*, **134,** 401 – 5
5. Forfar, J. O. and Nelson, M. M. (1973). Epidemiology of drugs taken by pregnant women: drugs that may affect the fetus adversely. *Clin. Pharmacol. Ther.*, **14,** 632 – 42
6. Lewis, P. (1983). Drug usage in pregnancy. In: Lewis, P. (ed.) *Clinical Pharmacology in Obstetrics*. (Boston: Wright – PSG)
7. *Physician's Desk Reference: 38th Edition* (1984). (Oradell, NJ: Medical Economics Company)

8. Boobis, A. R. and Lewis, P. J. (1983). Pharmacokinetics in pregnancy. In: Lewis, P. (ed.) *Clinical Pharmacology in Obstetrics,* (Boston: Wright – PSG)

9. Wood, S. M. and Hytten, F. E. (1981). The fate of drugs in pregnancy. *Clin. Obstet. Gynecol.,* **8,** 255 – 9

10. Rayburn, W. F. and Andresen, B. D. (1982). Principles of perinatal pharmacology. In: Rayburn, W. F. and Zuspan, F. (eds.) *Drug Therapy in Obstetrics and Gynecology.* (Norwalk, **CT:** Appleton – Century – Crofts)

11. Lewis, P. J. (1978). The effect of psychotropic drugs in the fetus. In: Sandler, M. (ed.) *Mental Illness in Pregnancy and the Puerperium,* (Oxford: Oxford University Press)

12. Werboff, J., Gottlieb, J., Dembicki, E. and Havlena, J. (1961). Postnatal effect of antidepressant drugs administered during gestation. *Exp. Neurol.,* **3:** 542 – 55

13. Werboff, J. and Kesner, R. (1963). Learning deficits of offspring after administration of tranquillizing drugs to the mothers. *Nature,* **197,** 106

14. Lewis, P. D., Patel, A., Bender, G. and Balazs, R. (1977). Do drugs acting on the nervous system affect all proliferation in the developing brain? *Lancet,* **1,** 399 – 401

15. Hill, H. F. and Engblom, J. (1984). Effects of pre- and postnatal haloperidol administrations to pregnant and nursing rats on brain catecholamine levels in their offspring. *Dev. Pharmacol. Ther.,* **7,** 188 – 7

16. Ordy, J. M., Samorajski, T. and Collins, R. L. (1966). Prenatal chlorpromazine effects on liver survival and behavior of mice offspring. *J. Pharmacol. Exp. Ther.,* **151,** 110 – 25

17. Golub, M. and Kornetsky, C. (1980). Seizure susceptibility and avoidance conditioning in adult rats treated prenatally with chlorpromazine. *Dev. Psychobiol.,* **7,** 79 – 88

18. Cooper, S. J. (1978). Psychotropic drugs in pregnancy: morphological and psychological adverse effects in offspring. *J. Biosoc. Sci.,* **10,** 321 – 34

19. Edlund, M. J. and Craig, T. J. (1984). Antipsychotic drug use and birth defects: an epidemiologic reassessment. *Comp. Psychol.,* **25,** 32 – 37

20. Goldberg, H. L. and DiMascio, A. (1978). Psychotropic drugs in pregnancy. In: Lipton, M. A., DiMascio, A. and Killam, K. F. (eds) *Psychopharmacology: A Generation of Progress* (New York: Raven Press)

21. Nurnberg, H. G. and Prudic, J. (1984). Guidelines for treatment of psychosis during pregnancy. *Hosp. Comm. Psychol.,* **35,** 67 – 71

22. Hill, R. M. and Stern, L. (1979). Drugs in pregnancy: effects on the fetus and newborn. *Curr. Therapeutics,* **20,** 131 – 50

23. Van Waes, A. and Van de Velde, E. J. (1969). Safety evaluation of haloperidol in the treatment of hyperemesis gravidarum. *J. Clin. Pharmacol,* **9,** 224

24. Hanson, G. W. and Oakley, G. P. (1975). Haloperidol and limb deformity. *J. Am. Med. Assoc.,* **231,** 26

25. Rawlings, W. J., Ferguson, R. and Maddison, T. G. (1963). Phenmetrazine and trifluoperazine. *Med. J. Aust.,* **1,** 370

26. Moriarity, A. J. and Nance, N. R. (1963). Trifluoperazine and pregnancy. *Can. Med. Assoc. J.,* **88,** 375 – 6

27. Stone, D., Siskind, V., Heinonen, O. P. *et al.* (1977). Antenatal exposure to the phenothiazines in relation to congenital malformations, perinatal mortality rate, birth weight, and intelligence quotient score. *Am. J. Obstet. Gynecol.,* **128,** 486 – 8

28. Rumeau-Rouquette, C., Goujard, J. and Huel, G. (1977). Possible teratogenic effects of phenothiazines in human beings. *Teratology,* **15,** 57

29. Milkovich, L. and Van den Berg, B. J. (1976). An evaluation of the teratogenicity of certain antinauseant drugs. *Am. J. Obstet. Gynecol.,* **125,** 244 – 8

30. Hannah, R. S., Roth, S. H. and Spira, W. (1982). The effects of chlorpromazine and phenobarbital on vasculogenesis in the cerebellar cortex. *Act. Neuropathol.* (Berl.), **57,** 306

31. Patel, A. J., Barochovsky, O., Borges, S. and Lewis, P. D. (1983). Effects of neurotropic drugs on brain cell replication in vivo and in vitro. *Monogr. Neurol. Sci.,* **9,** 99 – 110

32. Hannah, R. S., Roth, S. H. and Spira, A. W. (1982). The effects of chlorpromazine and phenobarbital on cerebellar purkinje cells. *Teratology,* **26,** 21 – 5

33. Rosengarten, H. and Friedhoff, A. J. (1979). Enduring changes in dopamine receptor cells of pups from drug administration to pregnant and nursing rats. *Science,* **203,** 1133 – 5

34. Robertson, R. T., Majka, J. A., Peter, C. P. and Bokelman, D. L. (1980). Effects of prenatal exposure to chlorpromazine on postnatal development and behavior of rats. *Toxicol. Appl. Pharmacol.*, **53**, 541 – 9

35. Hoffeld, D. R., NcNew, J. and Webster, R. L. (1968). Effect of tranquillizing drugs during pregnancy on activity of offspring. *Nature*, **218**, 357 – 8

36. Dallemagne, G. and Weiss, B. (1982). Altered adult behavior of mice following postnatal treatment with haloperidol. *Pharmacol. Biochem. Behav.*, **16**, 761 – 7

37. Hill, R. M., Desmond, M. M. and Kay, J. L. (1966). Extrapyramidal dysfunction in an infant of a schizophrenic mother. *J. Pediatr.*, **69**, 589

38. Desmond, M. M., Rudolph, A. J., Hill, R. M. *et al.* (1967). Behavioral alterations in infants born to mothers on psychoactive medication during pregnancy. In: Farrel, G. (ed.) *Congenital Mental Retardation*, (University of Texas, Austin)

39. Kris, E. B. (1965). Children of mothers maintained on pharmacotherapy during pregnancy and postpartum. *Curr. Ther. Res.*, **7**, 785 – 9

40. Tamer, A., McKey, R., Arias, D. *et al.* (1969). Phenothiazine induced extrapyramidal dysfunction in the neonate. *J. Pediatr.*, **75**, 479

41. Levy, W. and Wisniewsky, K. (1974). Chlorpromazine causing extrapyramidal dysfunction. *N. Y. St. Med. J.*, **74**, 684 – 5

42. O'Connor, M., Johnson, G. M. and Jamis, D. I. (1981). Intrauterine effects of phenothiazines. *Med. J. Aust.*, **1**, 416

43. Falterman, L. G. and Richardson, D. J. (1980). Small left colon syndrome associated with maternal ingestion of psychotropic drugs. *J. Pediatr.*, **97**, 300 – 10

44. Nielsen, J., Friedrich, U. and Tsubor, T. (1969). Chromosome abnormalities in patients treated with chlorpromazine, perphenazine, and lysergide. *Br. Med. J.*, **3**, 634 – 6

45. Gusdon, J. P. and Herbst, G. (1976). The effect of promethazine hydrochloride on fetal and maternal lymphocytes. *Am. J. Obstet. Gynecol.*, **126**, 730 – 1

46. Mason, C. G. (1977). Ocular accumulation and toxicity of certain systemically administered drugs. *J. Toxicol. Env. Health*, **2**, 977

47. Van Petten, G. R. (1975). Fetal cardiovascular effects of maternally administered tricyclic antidepressants, In: Morselli, P. L., Garatini, S. and Sereni, F. (eds). *Basic and Therapeutic Aspects of Perinatal Pharmacology*, (New York: Raven Press)

48. Barson, A. J. (1972). Malformed infants. *Br. Med. J.*, **2**, 45

49. McBride, W. G. (1972). Limb deformities associated with iminodibenzyl hydrochloride. *Med. J. Aust.*, **1**, 492

50. Idanpaan-Heikkila, J. and Saxen, L. (1972). Possible teratogenicity of imipramine/chloropyramine. *Lancet*, **2**, 282

51. Kuenssberg, E. V. and Knox, J. D. (1972). Imipramine in pregnancy. *Br. Med. J.*, **2**, 292

52. Sim, M. (1972). Imipramine and pregnancy. *Br. Med. J.*, **2**, 45

53. Crombie, D. L., Pinsent, R. J. and Fleming, D. (1972). Imipramine in Pregnancy. *Br. Med. J.*, **1**, 745

54. Scanlon, F. J. (1969). Use of antidepressant drugs during the first trimester. *Med. J. Aust.*, **2**, 1077

55. Jason, K. M., Cooper, T. B. and Friedman, E. (1981). Prenatal exposure to imipramine alters early behavioral development and beta adrenergic receptors in rats. *J. Pharmacol. Exp. Ther.*, **217**, 461

56. Coyle, I. R. (1975). Changes in developing behavior following prenatal administration of imipramine. *Pharmacol. Biochem. Behav.*, **3**, 799 – 807

57. Coyle, I. R. and Singer, G. (1975). The interactive effects of prenatal imipramine exposure and postnatal rearing conditions on behavior and histology. *Psychopharmacologia* (Berl.), **44**, 253 – 6

58. File, S. E. and Tucker, J. C. (1984). Prenatal treatment with clomipramine: Effects on the behavior of male and female adolescent rats. *Psychopharmacology*, **82**, 221 – 4

59. Dorner, G. (1975). Further evidence of permanent behavioral changes in rats treated neonatally with neurodrugs. *Endokrinologie*, **68**, 345 – 8

60. Dorner, G., Heicht, K. and Hinz, G. (1975). Teratopsychogenetic effects apparently produced by nonphysiological neurotransmitter concentrations during brain differentiation. *Endokrinologie*, **68**, 323 – 30

61. Dorner, G., Staudt, J., Wenzel, J. *et. al.* (1977). Further evidence of teratogenic effects

apparently produced by neurotransmitters during brain differentiation. *Endokrinologie,* **70,** 326 – 30

62. Schou, M., Amdisen, A. and Streenstrup, O. (1973). Lithium and pregnancy. II. Hazards to women given lithium during pregnancy and delivery. *Br. Med. J.,* **2,** 137

63. Wilbanks, G. D., Bressler, B., Peete, H. C. *et al.* (1970). Toxic effects of lithium carbonate in a mother and newborn infant. *J. Am. Med. Assoc.,* **213,** 856

64. Jefferson, J. W., Greist, J. H. and Ackerman, D. L. (1983). *Lithium Encyclopedia for Clincial Practice.* (Washington: American Psychiatric Press)

65. Szabo, K. T. (1970). Teratogenic effect of lithium carbonate in the fetal mouse. *Nature,* **225,** 73 – 5

66. Linden, S. and Rich, C. L. (1983). The use of lithium during pregnancy and lactation. *J. Clin. Psychiatry,* **44,** 358 – 61

67. Goldfield, M. D. and Weinstein, M. R. (1971). Lithium in pregnancy: a review with recommendations. *Am. J. Psychiatry,* **127,** 888 – 93

68. Schou, M., Goldfield, M. D., Weinstein, M. R. *et al.* (1973). Lithium and pregnancy – I. Report from the Register of Lithium Babies. *Br. Med. J.,* **2,** 135 – 6

69. Weinstein, M. R. and Goldfield, M. D. (1975). Cardiovascular malformations with lithium use during pregnancy. *Am. J. Psychol.,* **132,** 529 – 31

70. Hsu, J. M. and Rider, A. A. (1978). Effect of maternal lithium ingestion on biochemical and behavioral characteristics of rat pups. In: Johnson, F. N. and Johnson, S. (eds) *Lithium in Medical Practice,* (Baltimore: University Park Press)

71. Morrell, P. *et al.* (1983). Lithium toxicity in a neonate. *Arch. Dis. Child.,* **58,** 539 – 41

72. Schou, M. (1976). What happened later to the lithium babies? *Acta Psychiat. Scand.,* **54,** 193 – 7

73. Strothers, J. K., Wilson, D. W. and Royston, N. (1973). Lithium toxicity in a newborn. *Br. Med. J.,* **3,** 233 – 4

74. Woody, J. N., London, W. L. and Wilbanks, G. D. (1971). Lithium toxicity in a newborn. *Pediatrics,* **47,** 94 – 6

75. Wilson, N., Forfar, J. C. and Godman, M. J. (1983). Atrial flutter in a newborn resulting from maternal lithium ingestion. *Arch. Dis. Child.,* **58,** 538 – 9

76. Arnon, R. G., Marin-Garcia, J. and Peeden, J. N. (1981). Tricuspid valve regurgitation and lithium carbonate toxicity in a newborn infant. *Am. J. Dis. Child.,* **135,** 941 – 3

77. Karlsson, K., Linstedt, G., Lundberg, P. A. and Selstam, U. (1975). Transplacental lithium poisoning: reversible inhibition of fetal thyroid. *Lancet,* **1,** 1295

78. Mizrahi, E. M., Hobbs, J. and Goldsmith, D. (1979). Nephrogenic diabetes insipidus in transplacental lithium intoxication. *J. Pediatr.,* **94,** 493 – 5

9
Developmental Evaluation and Intervention for Drug-exposed Infants

KAYREEN A. BURNS

Infants born to chemically abusing mothers are at risk for deviations in behavioral and intellectual development, just as they are at risk for deviations in physical development. One of the major objectives of a perinatal addiction program is to assess the effects of intrauterine drug exposure on the developmental outcome of these infants. A second objective is to evaluate the psychological status of the mother, especially as that status may affect her relationship with her infant. These assessments of mother and child fulfill a twofold purpose:

1. They provide a clinical understanding of the psychological adjustments of the mother and child, which may become the basis for appropriate intervention.
2. They help to build a fund of research information on a high-risk group about whom we know very little.

The Northwestern Perinatal Services Project was established approximately 10 years ago to provide obstetric, pediatric and psychological services for pregnant addicted women and their offspring. When an infant is born to a woman enrolled in this project, the Neonatal Behavioral Assessment Scale[1] is administered. The BNBAS is designed to assess the neonate's capacity to organize interactive, motoric and arousal aspects of behavior in response to a structured series of examiner demands. With this instrument an initial observation may be made in a standardized fashion in order to estimate how well these compromised infants are making the transition from intrauterine to extrauterine environment. The BNBAS assumes that a normal newborn infant is already functioning at a very complex level, that he/she is equipped to defend himself from negative stimuli, and that he/she is able to organize internal control over interfering motor and autonomic reactions in order to attend to environmental stimuli[2]. Brazelton[3] notes that the BNBAS is sensitive to the neonate's ability to cope with both external and internal stimuli, and that the efficiency of this coping is reflected in the neonate's success at balancing internal stability with the intrusiveness of external stimulation. Since it has been demonstrated that narcotic-addicted infants are affected by their withdrawal for at least 6 months postpartum[4], many of the deviant responses obtained from these infants on the BNBAS are most likely caused by intrauterine drug exposure.

During an evaluation session using the BNBAS an examiner assesses the infant's ability to respond to a variety of stimuli as the infant moves from sleep through waking, fussiness, crying and full alertness. Scores are obtained for the infant's response to 20 reflex items used to estimate neurological intactness. There are 27 behavioral items used to assess the infant's interactive and motoric abilities, as well as capacity to organize state control and physiological responses to stress. Als[5] notes that the original purpose of the BNBAS was to assess individual differences among healthy fullterm newborns. However, since the 1970s the BNBAS has been used successfully to assess the effects of chemicals on the newborn, including obstetric medication and maternally ingested narcotics. The BNBAS is well suited to reveal the deficits in an infant's ability to organize a recovery from intrauterine exposure to drugs, and thereby an estimation may be made of the effect that such deficits may have on caretaking.

There is a normative range of response to the 27 behavioral items on the BNBAS, if they are administered while the infant is in one of the defined states of arousal assigned to each item. Interpretation of the normality of responses depends on the examiner's awareness of the infant's ability to move smoothly through the various levels of arousal (sleep, drowsy, alert, fussy or crying). Since the BNBAS is designed to guide an infant through a repertoire of these states, it is an excellent instrument to assess the deficits in state control in infants of drug-abusing mothers. The quality of an infant's ability to move from state to state provides an indicator of any CNS dysfunction which may be present. A normal infant expresses appropriate control by shutting out intrusive stimuli (response decrement), by taking in positive stimuli (alertness and orientation), and by modulating movements (motor maturity and tone). A normal infant also demonstrates some ability to organize tendencies to become under- or over-aroused, and therefore to achieve control over sudden environmental changes.

The BNBAS is administered at a halfway point between feedings in order to increase the likelihood that infants are comparable at the beginning of the assessment. Scores are based on the infant's optimal performance rather than typical performance as a way of controlling for the instability of infant behavior. Therefore an examiner is trained not only to score an infant's performance, but also to elicit optimal performance.

Data collected from the BNBAS serves a valuable research purpose, while the process of assessment serves a clinical purpose. At the Northwestern Perinatal Services Project the infant's mother is always present during the assessment. Following the evaluation the examiner discusses with the mother the specifics of her individual infant and suggests ways of interacting which will optimize their relationship. Mothers are encouraged to ask questions about their baby, about care-taking and development. The discussion is focused on the actual behaviors observed by the mother during the assessment, especially the infant's ability to remain in a sleep state during intrusive sights, sounds and touch, to take advantage of cuddling and handling, to visually focus and track and to respond to consoling successfully. Since most infants of drug-abusing mothers exhibit deficits in state control, mothers are advised about the extra help that such an infant will require in order to attain a semblance of organization. An attempt is made to help these mothers to recognize the infant's communication of stimulus overload, and even to be aware of some of the early indicators of impending distress (sneezing, averting, state change). The examiner uses modeling to teach methods of consoling (hand-holding, inhibition of movement, sucking). These mothers often express gratitude for this anticipatory guidance.

Despite significant doubts about the validity of the BNBAS[6], it is one of the most comprehensive instruments available for the study of newborn infants, and therefore provides the most enlightening information about the effect of maternal drug abuse on the newborn. Analyses of BNBAS scores have traditionally followed several routes. Als et al.[2] have criticized the item-by-item approach for several reasons:

1. most often authors do not hypothesize which items will differ;
2. so many items are involved that some differences may be due to chance alone; and
3. many of the items are related rather than independent, as many statistical procedures assume.

These authors recommend instead the use of typological and profile analysis which is used in most current studies[7].

At various points in the history of the Northwestern Perinatal Services Project researchers have analyzed the BNBAS data in order to gradually add to the fund of information about risk factors present in neonates who have been passively exposed to drugs. Results have demonstrated how these infants live their first days, weeks and months recovering from compromised fetal development and neonatal withdrawal. In the 1970s and early 1980s the majority of the women entering the project abused narcotics. Table 9.1 shows one of the first analyses of BNBAS data from this population. Infants were grouped according to type of drug use in the mothers (methadone, nonnarcotic polydrugs and nondrug use comparison controls). Mothers in Group I reported heroin use during conception and were placed on methadone maintenance by the end of the second trimester. Mothers in Group II used multiple licit or illicit nonnarcotic drugs throughout pregnancy. Mothers in Group III had no history of drug or alcohol use. All three groups were matched for the following maternal factors: race, maternal age, education, gravidity, prenatal care and nutrition. Significant differences were found in newborn infant responses

96

between all three groups on the BNBAS. Both drug groups had consolability, state lability, and predominant state scores significantly poorer than the control group. The methadone group obtained scores that were significantly different from both polydrug and control groups in items relating to visual and auditory orientation and motor maturity. These results indicate that neonatal addiction leads to compromised behavior both in methadone-addicted newborns and in infants whose mothers use nonnarcotic substances[8].

Table 9.1 Mean scores of BNBAS that discriminated between the groups

	Methadone (n=39)	Polydrug (n=19)	Drug-free (n=27)	
	$\bar{x}$***	$\bar{x}$	$\bar{x}$	p (Anova)
Visual inanimate orientation	3·25**	5·67	5·48	0·001
Auditory inanimate orientation	3·33*	5·55	5·19	0·001
Visual animate orientation	3·90**	4·91	5·65	0·01
Auditory animate orientation	3·86**	5·18	5·23	0·04
Motor maturity	3·26**	4·50	4·67	0·006
Consolability	4·52*	3·67*	6·50	0·001
Predominant state	4·13*	4·82*	3·96	0·02
State lability	3·13*	3·73*	1·63	0·001

*   Significant difference from drug-free
**   Significant difference from polydrug and drug-free
*** SD range from 0·4 to 2·4

Table 9.2 Mean scores of BNBAS items which discriminate between groups

	T and B (n=13)	Methadone (n=46)	Drug-free (n=27)	
	$\bar{x}$	$\bar{x}$	$\bar{x}$	p (Anova)
Interactive				
Inanimate visual orientation	5·2	3·3*	5·6	0·002
Inanimate auditory orientation	5·4	3·4*	5·3	0·001
Animate visual and auditory orientation	5·3**	5·0**	6·5	0·04
Motoric				
Motor maturity	4·7	3·2*	4·8	0·003
Babinski	2·3***	1·4	1·8	0·004
Automatic walking	1·5**	1·6**	2·0	0·002
Placing	1·4**	1·4**	1·9	0·006
Rooting	1·3	1·7	1·8	0·01
Organization, state				
Consolability	4·2**	4·4**	6·3	0·004
Predominant state	4·5***	4·1	3·9	0·04
Lability of state	3·3**	3·2**	1·6	0·001

*   Significant difference from drug-free and T and B
**   Significant difference from drug-free
*** Significant difference from drug-free and methadone
SD range from 0·1 to 2·7

Critics of the above study have noted that the pooling of a variety of nonopiate drug users into a polydrug group tends to confound the specific effects of individual drugs. This criticism led to the study of mothers using specific drugs. Table 9.2 shows a comparison made between a group of 13 infants whose mothers used pentazocine and tripelennamine (T's and blues) with a group of 46 methadone-addicted infants and a group of comparison controls[9]. Cluster score analysis of the BNBAS data revealed significantly poorer scores for both drug groups as compared to control subjects in regard to interactive ability. Infants of methadone-dependent mothers also showed significantly reduced motoric ability when compared to both controls and to the T's and blues group.

In Table 9.3 data are presented from a retrospective analysis in which scores from infants born to mothers who had been in the project since its beginning in 1976 were evaluated. Type of maternal drug use was divided into four categories: methadone, nonnarcotic sedative-stimulant, T's and blues and phenycyclidine (PCP). Means and standard deviations for those BNBAS items for which statistically significant differences were obtained are listed. All four groups showed significantly poorer consolability and lability of state, and significantly higher predominant state than the control group. The methadone group also showed significantly poorer orientation scores and motor maturity than any of the other drug groups.

Table 9.3 Mean scores of BNBAS items which discriminated between the groups*

	Methadone	Sedative/ stimulant	T & B	PCP	Drug-free
	(n=51)	(n=22)	(n=13)	(n=9)	(n=27)
	$\bar{x}$	$\bar{x}$	$\bar{x}$	$\bar{x}$	$\bar{x}$
Interactive					
Inanimate visual orientation	3·3*	5·7	5·2	6·0	5·6
Inanimate auditory orientation	3·4*	5·6	5·4	4·3	5·3
Animate visual orientation	3·9*	4·9	4·5	4·5	5·7
Animate auditory orientation	3·9*	5·2	4·3	4·5	5·2
Motoric					
Motor maturity	3·3*	4·5	4·7	5·0	4·8
Organization, state					
Consolability	4·4*	3·7*	4·2*	2·5*	6·3
Predominant state	4·1*	4·8*	4·5*	4·8*	3·9
Lability of state	3·2*	3·7*	3·3*	5·0*	1·6

*Anova (specific drug group × group V), $p<0.01$
SD range from 0·4 to 2·4

A more recent type of drug abuser to enroll at the perinatal project is the pregnant cocaine abuser. Over a 21-month period 23 cocaine-abusing women gave birth to infants who are being followed in the project. Twelve of these women were using cocaine only[10]. Table 9.4 lists the mean scores for the BNBAS items that discriminated between the cocaine group and a nondrug-using control group. When all 23 cocaine-exposed infants were grouped, they had a significantly greater number of startle and tremor responses than did the control infants. These results indicated that infants who were fetally exposed to cocaine had poor state control and poor interactive capabilities when compared to a comparison nondrug group. Many reflexive and motoric responses also showed significant differences. The cocaine-addicted newborns obtained poorer consolability scores as a group than any other group ever assessed in the project. These infants needed maximum intervention from the examiner to achieve even partial calming. This frequently required vigorous infant sucking and swaddling, hand-holding, and time out from examining.

Table 9.4   Mean BNBAS scores which discriminate cocaine group from drug-free group

	Cocaine (n=12) $\bar{x}$	Drug-free (n=15) $\bar{x}$
Inanimate visual orientation	3·0*	5·7
Inanimate auditory orientation	2·3*	5·5
Animate visual orientation	3·2*	5·9
Animate auditory orientation	2·8*	5·9
Animate visual and auditory orientation	3·7*	6·5
Ankle clonus	1·0*	1·9
Standing	1·4*	2·0
Automatic walking	1·2*	1·8
Moro reaction	2·2*	1·8
Motor maturity	4·2*	5·0
Pull to sit	5·5*	6·2
Consolability	2·3*	6·3
Lability of skin color	6·5*	3·1
Lability of states	4·6*	2·6

*Significant difference from drug-free group, $p < 0.02$
SD range from 0·5 to 2·6

SUMMARY

The findings of the studies completed in the Northwestern Perinatal Services Project have provided considerable information about the neonatal status of infants born to drug-abusing mothers. The studies cited above summarize most of the neonatal data published to date. The BNBAS has proved to be an effective instrument for providing clinical information to mothers, while at the same time it has been a comprehensive research procedure for gathering data about a pressing psychological issue. The findings of the Northwestern Project in regard to infants of narcotic-addicted mothers are similar to positive findings reviewed in articles by Householder et al.[11] and Jeremy and Hans[12]. However, the project has gone beyond the focus on a single type of drug, narcotics, and has added the whole new dimension for evaluating the effects of many types of drug dependencies during pregnancy. No other research projects have set out to clearly identify and classify pregnant drug-abusers in this fashion and then to analyze outcome data based on these classifications. These findings have documented that infants of all drug groups exhibit compromised developmental status as neonates. Infants born to cocaine-abusing women were the most compromised of infants during the neonatal period. However, the performance of infants born to methadone-addicted women was also affected significantly.

FOLLOW-UP DURING INFANCY

Infants enrolled in the Northwestern Perinatal Services Project are scheduled for appointments at regularly structured intervals. The instrument most often used to assess progress from 3 to 30 months of age is the Bayley Scales of Infant Development. Chasnoff et al.[13] have summarized the results of the Bayley Scale data (MDI and PDI) at 3, 6, 12 and 24 months) for two groups of drug-addicted newborns. Table 9.5 shows that no significant differences were obtained between the three groups (methadone, polydrug or controls) at any of the examination ages. The interpretation of these results is a bit difficult because there were so few subjects at the 12- and 24-month age periods. The results seem to indicate that these infants perform within normal limits when optimal testing conditions are used (one-to-one, highly structured setting with an experienced examiner and mother close by). In a follow-up study of children of methadone mothers Johnson et al.[14] discuss similar conclusions. Although there are many failed appointments in a clinic for this population, there is a tendency for mothers to be more motivated to bring their children back when their child experiences behavior difficulties in day-care, pre-school, or school settings. The complaints most often voiced by caretakers and teachers relate to attentional, motivational and behavioral deficits rather than learning deficits per se. The mechanisms behind these deficits and the way that they are related to intrauterine drug exposure are still unanswered research questions.

Table 9.5 Mean follow-up scores on the Bayley scales of infant development

		Methadone		Polydrug		Controls	
		Mean	n	Mean	n	Mean	n
3 months	MDI	105·0	31	106·7	19	99·2	34
	PDI	105·0	31	100·5	19	102·8	34
6 months	MDI	105·9	13	101·1	13	111·0	29
	PDI	103·9	13	105·0	13	107·6	29
12 months	MDI	104·2	11	104·8	8	105·8	27
	PDI	106·0	11	92·1	8	103·8	27
24 months	MDI	97·5	6	96·5	4	96·2	14
	PDI	99·3	6	100·5	4	98·2	14

Aylward[15] criticizes outcome studies such as that of Chasnoff et al.[13] and that of Johnson et al.[14]. He states that these studies fail to take into account issues that confound linear cause and effect relationships such as other drug use, sample selection, excessive dropout, obstetric and neonatal risk factors, and poor preconceptual nutrition. Matching cannot control for all these factors; therefore any conclusions from follow-up studies must be interpreted with caution.

It is widely accepted among follow-up researchers that developmental and intellectual scores do not offer adequate information about the deficits of these children. Data about the mother and her background often add a modum of meaning to data collected on the child. Mothers often bring with them to the delivery of the child, problems in personality, social resources and attitude[16].

THE BECK DEPRESSION INVENTORY

The Beck Depression Inventory (BDI) has been administered routinely as part of the intake assessment for pregnant women entering the Northwestern Perinatal Services Project. It is a self-report instrument which is designed to evaluate the extent and depth of depressive symptomology. Since it is a brief 13-item questionnaire it is easily collected from all women, and easily scored and interpreted according to norms established by the authors[17]. Burns et al.[18] have analyzed the first 54 BDIs collected from women entering the project. Table 9.6 gives the results of these BDIs as analyzed by age group. This drug-using group as a whole was more frequently depressed than the normal population. Over 50% of the drug-using women were moderately to severely depressed, according to their own report. Eight percent of the adolescent women scored in the depressive category, while 25% of the young adult women scored in this range. An astounding 60% of the older chemically dependent women obtained scores in the severely depressed range. These results are consistent with findings of other researchers[19,20].

Table 9.6 Summary of BDI scores by groups

	Teenagers		Young women		Older women		Total	
Mean BDI score	8·0		9·4		14·7		10.2	
BDI categories								
Normal (0–4)	3	(25%)	12	(43%)	1	(7%)	16	(30%)
Mild (5–7)	2	(17%)	3	(11%)	3	(20%)	9	(17%)
Moderate (8–15)	6	(50%)	5	(18%)	2	(13%)	12	(22%)
Severe (16+)	1	(8%)	7	(25%)	9	(60%)	17	(31%)
n	12		27		15		54	

A group of researchers in New Zealand[21] studied the relationship between family life events, child-rearing and maternal depression. They found that the relationship between family life events and problems in child-rearing is mediated by the severity of maternal depression. Women with many adverse life events suffered increased rates and severity of depression, which in turn resulted in higher rates of problems with child-rearing. It would seem to be the case in the women from the Northwestern Perinatal Services Project that the adverse life event, drug use, has resulted in increased levels of depression over the years. The expected final correlate is child-rearing problems.

ASSESSMENT OF MOTHER – CHILD RELATIONSHIP

A self-report instrument for the assessment of the mother and child's attitude and behavior toward one another is the Mother–Child Relationship Evaluation[22]. This is an experimental scale designed to establish a frame of reference for maternal attitudes toward her child. Responses to the 48 items can be clustered into four scales of maternal attitude: acceptance, overprotection, overindulgence and rejection. Preliminary date using this scale in the Northwestern Project indicate that scores on acceptance and rejection scales are within normal limits, whereas overprotection and overindulgence scales are elevated. It appears that these women are ambivalent about whether to be strict or lax in their parenting. Since both of these scales are elevated, it seems that the drug-addicted women are allowing the pendulum of parenting philosophy to swing from one extreme to the other. This confused oscillation between being overprotective and overindulgent probably reflects the women's own unstable personalities, and possibly the way that they were parented. At times they give their children everything indiscriminately as they would have wanted to have been treated, then at other times they become very authoritarian as they have seen other parents (maybe their own) behave under stress. When rigid parenting fails to meet their goals, they become angry, feel guilty, give up, and finally return to lax parenting again. This vicious cycle repeatedly occurs as long as outside intervention is un-available. By identifying such a parenting sequence through the use of the Mother – Child Relationship Evaluation such outside guidance may be offered to all mothers who are at risk for such problems. Guiding mothers to a more middle approach in their parenting has seemed to avoid some of the violent consequences of authoritarian styles and the behavior disorder consequences of lax parenting.

CASE STUDY

The following is an example of a mother – child dyad who have obtained project services for 4 years. The mother was 34 years of age when she enrolled in Perinatal Services. It was near the end of her second trimester, and she was placed on methadone maintenance for the remainder of her pregnancy. The infant was born at 40 weeks gestation and administered the Brazelton Scale at 2 days of age. Normal scores were obtained on response decrement items of the BNBAS, but the infant became irritable when uncovered. Even with the gentlest of handing for lower reflex items, she began to cry. Her full cry was very difficult to console, and some items could not be administered. A full alert state was never attained. In order to reduce irritability it was necessary to use tight swaddling, hand-holding and sucking on a pacifier.

The infant returned on a regular basis to a follow-up clinic. The following Mental and Psychomotor Developmental Indices were obtained on the Bayley Scales of Infant Development:

	Months of age					
	3	*6*	*9*	*12*	*24*	*30*
MDI	114	129	107	102	79	106
PDI	103	124	100	124	77	108

At 3 months of age the infant was very fragile and easily upset whenever the examiner attempted to focus the infant's attention. By 6 months of age the infant was able to sustain brief, but not yet normal, episodes of attention to task. At the 9-month exam attentional ability was somewhat better, but the infant had become abnormally active, although not aggressively active. The mother was aware of the deviancy in the activity level and was given suggestions for working on this problem. It was suggested that she guide the infant into calming activity and to avoid overstimulating situations. At the 12-month exam the infant was still extremely active and appeared to be driven to place any objects handled into her mouth. The significant drop in scores at 2 years of age may have been related to several factors. The child was extremely difficult to examine because of frequent refusal to cooperate and impulsive responding when cooperative. Verbal communication was limited to a few single-word utterances. By this time the mother had recognized that her child was difficult to care for, and she asked for help. The psychologist recommended a mother – child program that was designed to give mothers training in behavioral management. At the 30-month visit after 6 months of behavioral training, the child's attentional ability and behavior were much improved. During the exam she was happy and cooperative, following test instructions without hesitation. Her 30-month scores on the Bayley Scales reflected this behavioral improvement. The mother said that she could not keep going to the mother – child program and dropped out of the program before the trainers had recommended. When they returned to follow-up clinic for a 3-year assessment, some of the child's poor attending had returned. It took frequent refocusing of the child's attention and continuous reinforcement of cooperation from the examiner in order to help the child complete the required tasks on the Stanford – Binet Intelligence Scale. The mother found it very frustrating to hold her constantly squirming child on her lap during the evaluation. She had placed her child in a day-care center during the past few months. The director of the center had told her that the child was very difficult to keep focused on tasks, would wander away from group activities and walk around the center by herself. No aggressive behavior was reported. The mother expressed disappointment that the day-care center was unable to compensate for her own limited parenting skills. She described the mother–child relationship at home as two people living side-by-side without paying attention to each other.

On a self-report scale of development completed when the child was 4 years old, the mother responded in such a way that scores would have placed her child 6–12 months advanced for her age in all areas except language. Such exaggeration is a frequent experience when mothers in this project are asked to complete self-report measures. This scale included her rating of the child as advanced in social–emotional development despite the fact that a preschool teacher had recently reported significant immaturity, poor attentiveness and poor interactive ability with peers.

On the Mother–Child Relationship Scale completed at the 4-year visit deviant scores were obtained on the overindulgence, rejection and acceptance scales. On a home environment questionnaire the mother reported a significantly high frequency of aggression at home, as expressed in temper tantrums, depressive mood and vulnerability to upset. She also reported poor discipline, infrequently planned activities with her child, and in general infrequently talking to or playing with the child. These problems did not appear to be merely current developments, but had built up as an ongoing history of this mother – child relationship.

When the psychologist discussed these assessment findings with the mother, she said that she had been aware that their relationship was pathological. She expressed her dread of spending evenings at home with her child, and she especially hated the interaction that occurred at bedtime. Her approach has frequently been to allow her child to 'run until she drops', and then carries her off to bed. She described her frustration when she watches her child conform better to the demands of a young babysitter than to her own demands. She verbalizes her growing awareness that the day-care and preschool settings have not proved to be adequate substitutes for her own poor parenting skills. She worries that teachers may demand Ritalin to 'slow her down'. Any dependence on drugs to alter feelings reminds her of her own drug abuse that ultimately affected her child. The future is somewhat grim for this dyad. Each of the participants has brought problems to the relationship, and now it has become evident that the process of the relationship itself has become pathological.

This case study gives an example of the multi-factor aspect of outcome in children born of chemically abusing mothers. It also demonstrates that any single factor taken by itself is insufficient to produce the intensity of problems experienced. Rather it is the cumulative effect of a poor start on the mother – infant interaction, a poor start on environmental supports for proper cognitive and emotional development, a poor start on self-monitoring of state control and whatever other factors may be involved. Since so many of these factors negatively coincide in families of drug-abusers, it is no wonder that the general experience of clinicians is that long-term prognosis is poor. Only with longitudinal serial assessment, and immediate intervention, may we be confident that long-term change will occur.

REFERENCES

1. Brazelton, T. B. (1973). *Neonatal Behavioral Assessment Scale.* (Philadelphia: J. B. Lippincott)
2. Als, H., Tronick, E., Lester, B. and Brazelton, T. B. (1979). Specific neonatal measures: The Brazelton Neonatal Behavioral Assessment Scale. In Osofsky, J. D. (ed.) *Handbook of Infant Development,* pp. 185 – 215 (New York: John Wiley)
3. Brazelton, T. B. (1978). Introduction. In Sameroff, A. J. (ed.) Organization and stability of newborn behavior: a commentary on the Brazelton Neonatal Behavior Assessment Scale. *Monogr. Soc. Res. Child Dev.,* **43,** 1 – 13
4. Chasnoff, I. and Burns, W. (1984). The Moro reaction: a scoring system for neonatal narcotic withdrawal. *Dev. Med. Child Neurol.,* **26,** 484 – 9
5. Als, H. (1984). Newborn behavioral assessment. In Burns, W. and Lavigne, J. (eds) *Progress in Pediatric Psychology.* (Orlando: Grune & Stratton)
6. Sameroff, A. J. (1978). Summary and conclusions: the future of newborn assessment. In Sameroff, A. J. (ed.) Organization and stability of newborn behavior: a commentary on the Brazelton Neonatal Behavior Assessment Scale. *Monogr. Soc. Res. Child Dev.,* **43,** 102 – 17
7. Burns, K., Deddish, R., Burns, W. and Hatcher, R. (1983). Oscillating waterbeds: a demonstration of the effects of premature infant stimulation. *Dev. Psychol.,* **19,** 746 – 51
8. Chasnoff, I., Hatcher, R. and Burns, W. (1982). Polydrug- and methadone-addicted newborns: a continuum of impairment? *Pediatrics,* **70,** 210 – 13
9. Chasnoff, I., Hatcher, R., Burns, W. and Schnoll, S. (1983). Pentazocine and Tripelennamine ('T's and Blues'): effects on the fetus and neonate. *Dev. Pharmacol. Therapeutics,* **6,** 162 – 9
10. Chasnoff, I., Burns, W., Schnoll, S. and Burns, K. (1985). Cocaine use in pregnancy. *N. Engl. J. Med.,* **313,** 666 – 9
11. Householder, J., Hatcher, R., Burns, W. and Chasnoff, I. (1982). Infants born to narcotic-addicted mothers. *Psychol. Bull,* **92,** 453 – 68
12. Jeremy, R. and Hans, S. (1985). Behavior of neonates exposed in utero to methadone as assessed on the Brazelton Scale. *Infant Behav. Dev.,* **8,** 323 – 36
13. Chasnoff, I., Schnoll, S., Burns, W. and Burns, K. (1984). Maternal nonnarcotic substance abuse during pregnancy: effects on infant development. *Neurobehav. Toxicol. Teratol.,* **6,** 277 – 80
14. Johnson, H., Diano, A. and Rosen, T. (1984). 24-Month neuro-behavioral follow-up of children of methadone-maintained mothers. *Infant Behav. Dev.,* **7,** 115 – 23
15. Aylward, G. (1982). Methadone outcome studies: is it more than the methadone? *J. Pediatr.,* **101,** 214 – 15
16. Jeremy, R. and Hans, S. (1985). Behavior of neonates exposed in utero to methadone assessed on the Brazelton Scale. *Infant Behav. Dev.,* **8,** 323 – 36
17. Beck, A. and Beck, R. (1972). Screening depressed patients in family practice: a rapid technic. *Postgrad. Med.,* **52,** 81 – 5
18. Burns, K., Melamed, J., Burns, W., Chasnoff, I. and Hatcher, R. (1985). Chemical dependence and clinical depression. *J. Clin. Psychol.,* **41,** 851 – 4
19. Reynolds, W. and Gould, W. (1981). A psychometric investigation of the standard and short form Beck Depression Inventory. *J. Consult. Clin. Psychol.,* **49,** 306 – 7
20. Regan, D., Rudranff, and Finnegan, L. (1980). Parenting abilities in drug dependent women: the negative effects of depression. *Pediatr. Res.,* **14,** 454
21. Fergusson, D., Horwood, L. and Shannon, F. (1984). Relationship of family life events, maternal depression, and child-rearing problems. *Pediatrics,* **73,** 773 – 6
22. Roth, M. (1980). *The Mother – Child Relationship Evaluation Manual.* (Los Angeles: Western Psychological Services)

10
Psychopathology of Mother–Infant Interaction

WILLIAM J. BURNS

A human fetus is yoked to its mother in a nurturant bond in order to obtain the nutrients necessary for growth and development. However, it is through this same avenue that come substances which place the unborn infant at risk for disorders of growth and development. Alcohol, narcotics and other drugs are known to cross the placental barrier and to cause potentially injurious effects in the development of the embryo and fetus.

After birth has occurred the human infant is linked to the mother in an affectional bond that is meant to supply for both mother and infant the psychological nurturance necessary for them to grow and develop together[1]. If either or both mother and infant begin this relationship with deficits that place the relationship at risk for dysfunction, then not only is the dyadic relationship vulnerable to pathological interaction but also the individual outcome of each member of the dyad is at risk for pathology.

Relational difficulties between mother and infant do not always deserve to be labeled as pathology. The sequelae of many parenting difficulties are not long-lasting or intense enough to be called 'pathological', despite the considerable upset that may occur in the short term. For instance, some temporary problems with infant sleeping, eating or irritability may often be remedied with brief intervention. There are some problems which do become chronic, however, with adverse consequences for the relationship. This is potentially the case for the interactional relationship between infants and their chemically dependent mothers.

A complex of factors may be included in the causal chain which produces such a dysfunction, including: the withdrawal of the infant from intrauterine addiction[2–4], the ineptness of the mother[2,5], lack of personal resources for the parent[6,7], low socioeconomic status and maternal personality deviancies which lead to poor choices of lifestyle[8]. There is broad acceptance that a high risk for dysfunction exists in dyads where the mother is a chemical abuser. The question seems to be: what are the causes?

106

The Northwestern Perinatal Services Project[9] has attempted to research those prenatal variables[10], neonatal variables[11], and follow-up variables[12] which might relate to poor interactional functioning. It has been found that infants' interactive abilities may be composed differentially depending on the type of chemical abuse by the mother[11,13,14]. Special difficulties have been uncovered in the case of infants whose mothers use nonnarcotic drugs[15], especially cocaine[16].

INFANT CHARACTERISTICS

Withdrawal

There is a consensus[8] that infants born to mothers addicted to narcotics usually show characteristic signs of acute withdrawal within 24 – 48 hours after delivery, and improve somewhat after a few days. However, some infants show a pattern of improvement followed by a relapse at 2–4 weeks. A third pattern of withdrawal has also been noted in some infants who do not develop withdrawal symptoms until 2–3 weeks after delivery[17]. Symptoms of neonatal abstinence include disturbances of sleep, crying, sucking, feeding, activity level, and muscle tone.

This acute neonatal withdrawal is the drug-addicted mother's first experience in her relationship with her child, a type of relationship pathology that is common to drug-addicted mothers. Potentially a skilled mother could adjust to such a pathological condition, but not without great difficulty. As for unskilled mothers, the difficulties increase a great deal[18].

It has been well documented that normal mothers respond to changes in their normal infant's behavioral states[19]. Studies using the Brazelton Neonatal Behavioral Assessment Scale (BNBAS)[20] during the period of withdrawal have shown the abnormal behavioral states and interactional behaviors of infants of chemically dependent mothers[8,21]. There is no doubt that such interactional deficits are part of the causal chain which increases the risk of dysfunction in the mother – child interaction. Jeremy and Hans have noted that behaviors measured by the BNBAS during the first month of life are 'determinants' of the manner in which the mother and father will understand and relate to their child[21].

However, contrary to the opinion of these same authors that the differences in neurobehavior functioning between the narcotic exposed and control infants 'have largely disappeared by one month' (ref. 21, p. 333), Chasnoff and Burns[22] have identified a second period of withdrawal, a chronic period of deficient responsiveness to stimulation. In a longitudinal study of the neurobehavioral sequelae of methadone withdrawal Chasnoff and Burns found significant differences between methadone-exposed and comparison infants through the first 6 months of life.

Korner[23] has gathered evidence to show that the state of arousal level of a normal infant has a profound effect on the way that the mother treats her infant. In the case of abnormal infants there is even more pronounced evidence that deviant state control is a causal factor in the genesis of deviant mothering. Korner cites a study by Brazelton[24] whereby an infant with abnormal state control so demoralized the mother that she became depressed and totally ineffectual.

In summary, therefore, there is sufficient evidence to establish that infants born to chemically addicted mothers are at increased risk for interactional pathology.

MATERNAL CHARACTERISTICS

When correlational methods are used to detect dysfunction in a dyadic relationship, one is not justified in asserting that either member of the dyad is the cause of the dysfunction. For instance, Field[25] reported that in a sample of depressed mothers, the depression was often 'mirrored' in the infants' depressive-like behaviors. However, in another study of depressed mothers Brazelton[24] demonstrated that such depression may be a result of the struggle of a mother to care for an infant with deviant state patterns.

There are some maternal dimensions that are more convincing than others as causal factors in poor maternal–infant interaction. For instance, Csofsky and Connors[26] have pointed out the important contributions of social class differences and maternal attitudes and perceptions in the quality of mother–infant interaction. Massie[27] has shown the significant influence of parental emotional adjustment on mother–infant interaction by filming sequences in which there is a progressive deterioration in infant responsiveness as a direct result of aberrant interactive behavior on the part of the mother.

In the case of women who are chemical abusers, it is assumed that in most instances their use of drugs during pregnancy is not a temporary experimentation with drugs, but an enduring pathological dependence. If indeed their chemical abuse is a part of a consistent maladaptive lifestyle, then their personality disorder places these mothers at high risk for associated problems such as mood and character disturbances[28]. In the Northwestern Memorial Hospital sample of substance-abusing mothers, significant mood disturbances have been found through the use of self-report measures such as the Beck Depression Scale[29]. Significant personality disturbances have also been uncovered in the form of sexual abuse[30]. In another sample of methadone-maintained pregnant women, Regan et al.[31] found a very high frequency of violence in the lives of these women. Many were beaten as children by their mothers, and beaten as adults by their spouses, as well as molested and raped. Kaltenbach et al.[32] found this same group of women to be significantly lacking in ordinary knowledge about child development.

A typical case of a drug abusing mother is the following example from the Northwestern Perinatal Services program.

This is a two-parent family into which the infant was born while the mother was using methadone as prescribed in the detoxification program. The mother was in her late twenties, a high school drop-out and unemployed. Evaluation with the Beck Depression Scale showed a moderate elevation of self-reported depression.

On the Brazelton Scale given during the first 2 weeks after delivery, her infant exhibited mildly increased muscle tone in the legs, decreased ability to visually track an object, and difficulty maintaining balanced state control. By 4 weeks of age some of these findings had improved, but a follow-up evaluation at 3 months of age using the Bayley Scales of Infant Development showed considerable delay in both mental and psychomotor development. At that time the mother reported considerable difficulty relating to the infant because of the child's continued irritability. On a self-report scale regarding the mother– child relationship this mother rated herself to be below average in both overprotectiveness and overintrusion in the relationship.

The above difficulties occurred despite the fact that this mother had received intervention in the form of counseling and education concerning ways to deal with these very problems. It seems that, although educational counseling may help somewhat, this method of intervention offers an incomplete solution for such an intense problem.

Neither is it fair to use the mother as a scapegoat, or to label her as 'predictor'. Outcries against mother-blaming[33] have forced researchers of early social development to orient more of their attention to the infant and the father.

FAMILY CHARACTERISTICS

Normal family dynamics place considerable demands on the parents and children to cope with any special problems that arise[34]. When a new child is born, the father not only relates directly with the newborn infant, but also has indirect effects on the infant by affecting the mother's attitude toward herself and toward the infant[35]. It is considered to be a significant loss when the father is absent or psychologically unsupportive[7]. Thus, the scenario necessary for normal mother–infant interaction presumes the presence of a supportive father and husband.

In the case of a physical condition, such as drug withdrawal, which has a significant impact on the child's psychological adjustment, there will be considerable demands placed on the coping abilities of the family[36]. As in the case of any crisis, the perception by parents that a disorder is present is the signal for anxiety concerning their own hopes for future happiness and security as a family. These expectations develop for both parents during the mother's pregnancy. Among pregnant mothers who have been using drugs it is especially common for them to begin worrying about their infant's condition even before the birth of the infant. Having heard from other mothers about the withdrawal facing the infant at birth, a sense of personal guilt may develop during the last months of pregnancy. Parallel with the development of guilt and anxiety about the suffering they will have caused the infant, these mothers commonly attempt to cope by denying the existence of the problem. They fantasize that their infant will escape withdrawal.

Thus, even before the infant is born, there may be a climate of anxiety, guilt and nonacceptance of the severity of the infant's condition. Such a climate increases the risk not only of rejecting the accuracy of the diagnosis of neonatal withdrawal, but also the rejection of the infant, and in turn, such a maladjustment can lead to the mother's failure to provide proper care for the specialized needs of her infant during withdrawal and become part of the causal chain in the production of pathology in the mother–infant relationship. The presence of a supportive father during this crisis would provide a positive coping force to stem the tide of dysfunction between mother and child. The importance of including an analysis of the effect of paternal interaction in such a case has been shown by Lamb and Elster[37].

For many infants of drug-abusing mothers there is no father in the home. Even in the case where the father is present, the relationship between mother and father may be unstable, or the birth of an infant with problems may lead to destabilization of an already tenuous relationship. A vicious downward cycle of family interaction may occur with crises other than that of an infant born in chemical withdrawal, but in few cases are the dynamics of the pathology so clear. Such a process may end with the total isolation of the mother from all social resources, a situation which would be very risky for the infant when the mother–infant relationship deteriorates and allows for extremes of pathology such as the cases of neonatal sexual abuse found in the NMH program[30].

In these cases of abuse (fellatio) the mothers began regular sexual molestation of their sons as newborns and continued through the second year of life. They were all women who lived alone and had no steady male relationship. Some of them had experienced sexual abuse themselves, and most of them had sexual identity problems. On psychiatric examination they had all previously been diagnosed as 'borderline personalities'. This neonatal incest is an example of the most pathological type of adjustment that may occur in the mother–infant relationship. The fact that such a rarely occurring pathology could happen with such frequency in this population, is further evidence for the high potential for the occurrence of pathology in the mother–infant relationship.

DEVELOPMENT OF THE MATERNAL–INFANT INTERACTION

The neonatal period

Critical periods of interactional development have gradually come to light as a result of recent research findings. It is obvious that infants undergoing withdrawal are hindered from attaining these social milestones in a normal fashion. Tronick has emphasized the elements of affectivity and sharing as essentials for the proper development of interactive capability. Instead of conceptualizing the mother–infant interaction as mainly mother-directed or infant-directed, the interaction is viewed as a co-creation of each member of the dyad as the two are in the state of interacting. Interacting is a state of co-orientation in which the focus of attention of both partners may well be on a third object[38]. An infant who is experiencing chemical withdrawal has little energy for spontaneous engagement with animate or inanimate objects[16]. Therefore these infants miss many of the formative aspects of this earliest period of interactive development.

Infancy

With the advent of abilities to reach and grasp, the importance of an accurately functioning motor system becomes primary in the mother–infant interaction. Since the motor system in infants of drug-abusing mothers has been found to be deficient[7], the primary mode of interaction at this age level is at high risk for dysfunction.

Toddlerhood

Language development is the final step in the acquisition of communication skills needed for human interaction. Blatman and Lipsitz[39] found that when problems developed in the children of drug-abusing mothers, who were over 2 years of age, these problems were primarily speech and language disorders and perceptual problems.

Therefore, at each stage of interactional development the infants and children of drug-abusing mothers have demonstrated deficiencies that coincide with behaviors normally expected to produce interactive progress at each stage. These children are thus at risk for cumulative deficits in social interaction during each successive stage of their entire early developmental period.

DIRECT OBSERVATION OF INTERACTION

The study of parent–infant interaction has been carried out in the form of case studies[40], retrospective case–control studies[8], anterospective and prospective studies. Analyses have been performed using frequencies of discrete behaviors, durations of behavior, derived measures of behavioral frequencies and correlations of frequencies and derived measures[41] as well as times series analyses[42] including conditional probabilities for the concurrence of behaviors[43], lag sequential analysis[44] and cycles of behavioral units[45]. Analyses have used ratings of such dimensions as attachment[46], rearing competence[47] and a variety of other interactional dimensions[48].

Yarrow and Anderson[49] in a critique of procedures for studying mother–infant interaction have noted that no one strategy for observing and recording parent–infant interaction is, in itself, preferable to any other strategy. In fact, Kaye[50] argues that it is only when microanalytic techniques are combined with macroanalytic methods that dyadic dialogue can be understood. It is safe to conclude that, if we are to understand the complexities of interactive failure in infants and their chemically abusing mothers, many strategies of direct observation need to be systematically applied.

Currently, of drug-abusing mothers and their infants, only one study using direct observation of the interaction has been published in a refereed journal. In that study Jeremy and Bernstein[7] found that rating of the infant's interactive capability in these dyadic situations was primarily related to the examiner's ratings of activity level and tension on the Bayley Infant Behavior Record. The mother's interactive capability as rated on a scale of mothering was most dependent on the mother's IQ score, years of schooling, severity of psychopathology, and stability of her relationship with the father. It was the opinion of these researchers that narcotic use was only one of a complex of risk factors affecting the mother–infant interactions of this population. In another study Householder[51] found that, compared to matched controls, evaluation of mother–infant interactions in dyads in which the mother was addicted to narcotics showed significant behavioral indicators of interactional dysfunction.

In general the study of mother–infant interactions has taken place within the context of normal parenting and normal infant development[52] or in the context of separation and attachment[53]. Relatively little research has been done on interaction where the mother or infant has an identified disorder[27,54,55] or on the disordered interaction itself[56]. Although almost no research has been done on the relationship between infants and their drug-abusing mothers, there is little doubt that the potential for dysfunction is quite high for dyads in which the mother is chemically dependent.

In the present review several causal factors have been discussed which are potentially involved in the development of a pathological relationship between mother and child.

1. Infant withdrawal creates extra stress on the process of child-rearing, which makes it very difficult for the mother to distinguish the infant's personal distress from its increasing attempts to communicate. Abnormal state control and deficits in motor and orientation abilities make these infants poor interactional partners.
2. Drug-abusing mothers have an increased frequency of mood disorders and are at risk for the development of character disturbances, which have been shown to include abuse of their infants. Such a tendency towards personal and social instability makes many of these mothers poor interactional partners.
3. The environments in which these infants and mothers are found to relate often include the absence of a father or the presence of a psychologically unsupportive father. Often these mother–infant dyads are isolated from all relatives and friends. The unemployed mother, left alone to brood about an unsuccessful relationship with a newborn infant, may easily fall into even more deviant forms of mother–infant interaction such as neonatal incest.

Research thus far has offered only a few hints regarding the dynamics of these three potential causes of mother–infant interactional pathology. Until such time as these dynamics are better defined we are left with the imperative to intervene. Several authors have made suggestions about the intervention with infants and mothers at risk for interactional pathology. Bradley-Johnson[57] has discussed the use of psychological assessment with infants as a form of intervention and parent education. Considerable expertise is required in both evaluation and intervention in order to effectively provide such a service for parents. The benefits of such an approach include:

1. helping parents to be more realistic about the behaviors which they may expect from their infant,
2. providing a concrete model of interaction with the infant, and
3. motivating parents to look for similar responses from their infant at home.

Whether parents are seen as part of a group or as individuals, it seems necessary for them to learn more about child development and to understand how different parenting behaviors may lead to rather predictable outcomes in their child. Facilitating mother–child relationships may be not only a matter of educating these mothers in child development, social discourse and communication, but in giving them concrete roles to guide their parenting behavior.

Clark and Seifer[58] have offered a list of such roles including the following:

1. The responsibility for initiating interaction usually belongs to the adult in the early stages of infancy.
2. It is also up to the adult to make sure that the infant is allowed time to take his or her turn in responding.
3. Both mother and infant must gradually learn to speak the same language, to be sensitive to each other's signals (no matter how subtle) and to let each other know when they are responding to such signals.

Even after these rules have been understood, parents may need help complying with such roles. The parenting of a high-risk infant requires an adjustment above and beyond that required of a parent of a normal infant. Kaye[59] notes that good parenting requires a certain amount of pretense in order to lead their offspring to an appropriate goal. It takes courage and expertise to be a parent. In the face of pathology in the parent–child relationship it would take considerable motivation and understanding to reverse such a trend, especially at a later age.

REFERENCES

1. Tronick, E. (1982). Affectivity and sharing. In Tronick, E. (ed.) *Social Interchange in Infancy: Affect, Cognition and Communication*, pp. 1 – 6. (Baltimore: University Park Press)
2. Finnegan, L. P. and Macnew, B. A. (1974). Care of the addicted infant. *Am. J. Nurs.,* **74,** 685 – 93
3. Finnegan, L. P. (1979). Pathophysiological and behavioral effects of the transplacental

113

transfer of narcotic drugs to be foetuses and neonates of narcotic-dependent mothers. *Bull. Narc.,* **31,** 1 – 58

4. Kron, R. E., Finnegan, L. P., Kaplan, S. L., Litt, M. and Phoenix, M. D. (1975). The assessment of behavioral change in infants undergoing narcotic withdrawal: comparative data from clinical and objective methods. *Addict. Dis.,* **2,** 257 – 75
5. Wilson, G. S., McCreary, R., Kean, J. and Baxter, J. (1979). The development of preschool children of heroin-addicted mothers: a controlled study. *Pediatrics,* **63,** 135 – 41
6. Belsky, J. and Vondra, J. (1985). Characteristics, consequences and determinants of parenting. In L'Abate, L. (ed.) *The Handbook of Family Psychology and Therapy*, vol. 1, pp. 523 – 56. (Homewood, Ill.: Dorsey Press)
7. Jeremy, R. J. and Bernstein, V. J. (1984) Dyads at risk: methadone-maintained women and their four-month-old infants. *Child Dev.,* **55,** 1141 – 54
8. Householder, J., Hatcher, R., Burns, W. and Chasnoff, I. (1982) Infants born to narcotic addicted mothers. *Psychol. Bull.,* **92,** 453 – 67
9. Rosner, M., Keith, L. and Chasnoff, I. (1982) The Northwestern University Drug Dependence Program: the impact of intensive prenatal care on labor and delivery outcomes. *Am. J. Obstet. Gynecol.,* **144,** 23 – 7
10. Keith, L., Panio, A., Filstead, W., DiMenza, G. and London, P. (1979) The effects of maternal drug addiction on fetal growth and development. In *Proceedings of the First International Congress of Auxology*, pp. 521–9. (Milan, Italy: Centro Auxologico Italiano di Piancavallo)
11. Chasnoff, I., Hatcher, R. and Burns, W. (1982) Polydrug- and methadone-addicted newborns: a continuum of impairment? *Pediatrics,* **70,** 210 – 13
12. Chasnoff, I., Hatcher, R. and Burns, W. (1980) Early growth patterns of methadone-addicted infants. *Am. J. Dis., Child.,* **134,** 1049 – 51
13. Chasnoff, I., Hatcher, R., Burns, W. and Schnoll, S. (1983). Pentazocine and Tripelennamine ('T's and Blue's): effects of the fetus and neonate. *Dev. Pharmacol. Ther.,* **6,** 162 – 9
14. Chasnoff, I., Burns, W., Hatcher, R. and Burns, K. (1983). Phencyclidine: effects on the fetus and neonate. *Dev. Pharmacol. Ther.,* **6,** 404 – 8
15. Chasnoff, I., Schnoll, S., Burns, W. and Burns, K. (1984) Maternal nonnarcotic substance abuse during pregnancy: effects on infant development. *Neurobehav. Toxicol. Teratol.,* **6,** 277 – 80
16. Chasnoff, I., Burns, W., Schnoll, S. and Burns, K. (1985). Cocaine use in pregnancy. *N. Engl. J. Med.,* **313,** 666 – 9
17. Cloherty, J. (1980). Drug withdrawal. In Cloherty, J. and Stark, A. (eds) *Manual of Neonatal Care*, pp. 15 – 18. (Boston: Little Brown)
18. Davis, M. and Shanks, P. (1975). Neurological aspects of perinatal narcotic addiction and methadone treatment. *Addict. Dis.,* **2,** 203 – 26
19. Papousek, H. and Papousek, M. (1977) Mothering and the cognitive head-start: psychological considerations. In Schaffer, H. R. (ed.) *Studies in Mother–Infant Interactions*, pp. 63 – 85. (London: Academic Press)
20. Brazelton, T. B. (1973) *Neonatal Behavioral Assessment Scale.* (Philadelphia: J. B. Lippincott)
21. Jeremy, R. J. and Hans, S. L. (1985) Behavior of neonates exposed in utero to methadone as assessed on the Brazelton Scale. *Infant Behav. Dev.,* **8,** 323 – 36
22. Chasnoff, I. and Burns, W. (1984). The Moro reaction: a scoring system for neonatal narcotic withdrawal. *Dev. Med. Child. Neurol.,* **26,** 484 – 9
23. Korner, A. (1974) The effect of the infant's state, level of arousal, sex, and ontogenetic stage on the caregiver. In Lewis, M. and Rosenblum, L. (eds) *The Effect of the Infant on its Caregiver*, pp. 105 – 22. (New York: John Wiley)
24. Brazelton, T. (1961) Psychophysiologic reactions in the neonate. I. The value of observation of the neonate. *J. Pediatr.,* **58,** 508 – 17
25. Field, T. (1984) Early interactions between infants and their postpartum depressed mothers. *Infant Behav. Dev.,* **7,** 517 – 22
26. Osofsky, J. and Connors, K. (1979) Mother – infant interaction: an integrative view of a complex system. In Osofsky, J. (ed.) *Handbook of Infant Development*, pp. 519 – 48. (New York: John Wiley)

27. Massie, H. N. (1982) Affective development and the organization of mother–infant behavior from the perspective of psychopathology. In Tronick, E. (ed.) *Social Interchange in Infancy: Affect, Cognition and Communication*, pp. 161–182. (Baltimore: University Park Press)

28. American Psychiatric Association (1980) *Diagnostic and Statistical Manual of Mental Disorders*, 3rd edn. (Washington, DC: American Psychiatric Association)

29. Burns, K., Melamed, J., Burns, W., Chasnoff, I. and Hatcher, R. (1986) Chemical dependency and depression in pregnancy. *J. Clin. Psychol.* (In press)

30. Chasnoff, I., Burns, W., Schnoll, S., Burns, K., Chism, G. and Kyle-Spore, L. (1984) Maternal/neonatal incest. *Pediatr. Res.*, **18,** 173

31. Regan, D., Leifer, B. and Finnegan, L. (1982) Generations at risk: Violence in the lives of pregnant drug abusing women. *Pediatr. Res.*, **16,** 91 (abstr. 77)

32. Kaltenbach, K., Leifer, B. and Finnegan, L. (1982). Knowledge of child development in drug dependent mothers. *Pediatr. Res.*, **16,** 87 (abstr. 52)

33. Caplan, P. J. and Hall-McCorguodale, I. (1985). The scapegoating of mothers: a call for a change. *Am. J. Orthopsychiatry*, **55,** 610 – 13

34. Dunn, J. and Munn, P. (1985) Becoming a family member: family conflict and the development of social understanding in the second year. *Child Dev.*, **56,** 480 – 92

35. Parke, R. D. (1979) Perspectives on father–infant interaction. In Osofsky, J. (ed.) *Handbook of Infant Development*, pp. 549 – 90. (New York: John Wiley)

36. Lavige, J. and Burns, W. (1981) *Pediatric Psychology* (New York: Grune & Stratton)

37. Lamb, M. and Elster, A. (1985) Adolescent mother–infant–father relationships. *Dev. Psychol.*, **21,** 768 – 73

38. Collis, G. (1977) Visual co-orientation and maternal speech. In Schaffer, H. R. (ed.) *Studies in Mother – Infant Interaction*, pp. 355 – 75. (London: Academic Press)

39. Blatman, S. and Lipsitz, P. J. (1972) Children of women maintained on methadone: accidental methadone poisoning of children. *Proceedings of the 4th National Conference on Methadone Treatment*, **4,** 175 – 6

40. Mintzer, D., Als, H., Tronick, E. and Brazelton, T. (1985) Parenting an infant with a birth defect: the regulation of self esteem. *Zero to Three*, **5,** 1 – 8

41. Hinde, R. and Herrmann, J. (1977) Frequencies, durations, derived measures and their correlations in studying dyadic and triadic relationships. In Schaffer, H. R. (ed.) *Studies in Mother–Infant Interaction*, pp. 19 – 46. (London: Academic Press)

42. Gottman, J. and Ringland, J. (1981) The analysis of dominance and bidirectionality in social development. *Child Dev.*, **52,** 393 – 412

43. Brown, J., Bakeman, R., Synder, R., Fredrickson, W., Morgan, S. and Hepler, R. (1975) Interactions of black inner-city mothers with their newborn infants. *Child Dev.*, **46,** 677 – 86

44. Sackett, G. (1979). The lag-sequential analysis of contingency and cyclicity in behavioral interaction research. In Osofsky, J. (ed.) *Handbook of Infant Development*, pp. 623 – 52. (New York: John Wiley)

45. Lester, B., Hoffman, J. and Brazelton, T. (1985). The rhythmic structure of mother–infant interaction in term and preterm infants. *Child Dev.*, **56,** 15 – 27

46. Beksky, J., Rovine, M. and Taylor, D. (1984). The Pennsylvania infant and family development project. III: The origins of individual differences in infant–mother attachment: maternal and infant contributions. *Child Dev.*, **55,** 718 – 28

47. McGowan, R. and Johnson, D. (1984). The mother–child relationship and other antecedents of childhood intelligence: a casual analysis. *Child Dev.*, **55,** 810 – 20

48. Field, T. (1980) Interactions of preterm and term infants with their lower- and middle-class teenage and adult mothers. In Field, T., Goldberg, S., Stern, D. and Sostek, A. (eds) *High Risk Infants and Children*, pp. 113 – 32. (New York: Academic Press)

49. Yarrow, L. and Anderson, B. (1979). Procedures for studying parent–infant interactions: a critique. In Thoman, E. (ed.) *Origins of the Infants' Social Responsiveness*, pp. 209 – 23. (Hillsdale, NJ: Lawrence Eulbam Associates)

50. Kaye, K. (1977). Toward the origin of dialogue. In Schaffer, H. R. (ed.) *Studies in Mother – Infant Interaction*, pp. 89 – 117. (London: Academic Press)

51. Householder, J. (1980) An investigation of mother–infant interaction in a narcotic-addicted population. Unpublished doctoral dissertation, Northwestern University

52. Schaffer, H. R. (1977) Early interactive development. In Schaffer, H. R. (ed.) *Studies in Mother – Infant Interaction*, pp. 3 – 16. (London: Academic Press)
53. Bretherton, I. (1985) Attachment theory: retrospect and prospect. In Bretherton, I. and Waters, E. (eds) Growing Points of Attachment Theory and Research. Monogr. Soc. Res. Child Dev., **50,** 3 – 25
54. Als, H. (1982) The unfolding of behavioral organization in the face of a biological violation. In Tronick, E. Z. (ed.) *Social Interchange in Infancy: Affect, Cognition and Communication,* pp. 125 – 60. (Baltimore: University Park Press)
55. Jones, O. H. (1977) Mother–child communication with pre-linguistic Down's syndrome and normal infants. In Schaffer, H. R. (ed.) *Studies in Mother–Infant Interaction,* pp. 379 – 402. (London: Academic Press)
56. Field, T. (1979) Interaction patterns of preterm and term infants. In Field, T., Sostek, A., Goldberg, S. and Shuman, H. (eds) *Infants Born at Risk,* pp. 333 – 56. (New York: SP Medical & Scientific Books)
57. Bradley-Johnson, S. (1982) Infant assessment as intervention and parent education. *Infant Ment. Health J.,* **3,** 293 – 7
58. Clark, G. and Seifer, R. (1983) Facilitating mother–infant communication: a treatment model for high-risk and developmentally-delayed infants. *Infant Ment. Health J.,* **4,** 67–82
59. Kaye, K. (1982) *The Mental and Social Life of Babies: How Parents Create Persons.* (Chicago: University of Chicago Press)

11
Methodologic Issues in Investigations of Drug Abuse in Pregnancy

ALICE O. MARTIN

Studies of drug abuse in pregnancy pose no problems different from those in other types of medical investigations; however, they are characterized by a specific subset of analytic and interpretive problems. Foremost among these are vague hypotheses and study designs, difficulties in finding appropriate controls, small sample sizes, and loss of patients to follow-up. These problems will be discussed and guidelines presented on how to avoid them or to minimize their impact. These guidelines should be helpful to those planning and implementing research strategies, as well as to those who must apply the conclusions of the research of others in caring for their patients or formulating public policy.

Table 11.1   Format for a medical investigation and report of results

I   What is the *hypothesis* being tested or the *objective* of the study?
II   What is the experimental design?
    A.   To which *reference target population* are results of study or a *sample* of patients or animals to apply?
    B.   What *type* of *study* is appropriate to answer the basic questions posed (hypothesis, objective)? (see Table 11.2).
    C.   Which *variables* will be determined? Which are *end point, response or outcome* variables? Which are *confounding variables*, those which may affect the outcome variable? What is their reliability and reproducibility?
    D.   What *sample size* is required to detect true differences that are large enough to be clinically relevant?
    E.   How will the data be collected? Will the study be double-blind? Randomized?
    F.   If *controls* are needed, how will they be selected to assure comparability with the *experimental* or *study* patients?
III   Are the data clearly presented?
    A.   Are numbers on graphs and tables internally consistent? Do they match those in the text?
    B.   Are the conclusions supported by the graphs and tables?
    C.   Are these constructed appropriately?
IV   Are the data appropriately *analyzed*?
    A.   Are assumptions of the tests fulfilled?
    B.   Are the tests appropriate for the type of variable? For the hypothesis or objective?
V   Are the conclusions supported by the data?

Table 11.1 outlines the ideal format of an investigation and its resultant publication.

1. THE HYPOTHESIS OR OBJECTIVE

The hypothesis or objective must be clearly and specifically defined *prior* to implementing a study design; otherwise the correct experimental design cannot be selected, and conclusions of the study may not be valid. The temptation to analyze data collected initially for descriptive purposes should be tempered by the knowledge that 'statistical tests of hypotheses are strictly applicable only to hypotheses fully and explicitly formed before the data are examined'[1]. This does not mean *a posteriori* hypotheses cannot be tested, but the inferences made from them are weak. Particularly to be avoided is the practice of singling out 'interesting -looking' outcome variables, comparing their frequency to that in some 'normal' group, and ignoring other variables. For example, because the birthweight of infants of heroin addicts may seem 'low', an investigator wishes to compare it to average birthweight of infants whose mothers were drug-free. The rules of chance on which statistical analyses are based are violated if only the unusual outcomes (those appearing different from normal) are selected for statistical analysis. The main function of interesting but unexpected observations is to generate hypotheses to be tested *in subsequent studies*. This protects against making too much of a chance finding that would not appear in a replicate study, yet permits likely etiologic factors to be ferreted out from a myriad of possibilities.

In order to be meaningful the hypothesis must not be so broad that it cannot be tested with a finite sample of patients and a reasonable investment of personnel and resources. Furthermore, the hypothesis should determine *a priori* what type of patients are included, what type of controls are needed to answer the question posed, and what type of statistical analysis is appropriate.

An example of a specific hypothesis would be: 'Infants of mothers on methadone maintenance during pregnancy have the same rates of perinatal mortality as do infants of drug-free mothers.' Another would be 'There is no difference in respiratory rate, blood pressure, and serum thyroxine levels of phenobarbital-treated infants compared to those on paregoric.' Notice that the hypothesis is phrased in terms of 'no difference' between groups of infants, even though the investigator may really be interested in, or expect, a difference. The 'null hypothesis' is phrased in terms of 'no difference', 'no association', or 'no improvement' in order to be able to apply statistical analysis. Statistical techniques are generally based on showing how likely it is that observations obtained in an investigation have occurred by chance if the null hypothesis is indeed true. This concept of the null hypothesis will be explained further in the section on statistical analysis.

An example of a hypothesis that is too vague would be: 'Methadone maintenance is harmful for pregnancy.' Is the mother or fetus the unit of study? What is 'harmful'? What outcomes will be studied? It is not sufficient to state the general topic of interest; specific hypotheses must precede study design formulation; otherwise, in the example stated above, data might be collected on numerous variables recorded during and after pregnancy. The investigator would then search to see if anything looked 'harmful' to him, and focus his conclusions and analysis accordingly. This ignores the implicit comparisons of other variables on which data were collected. 'Positive' results are almost guaranteed by this approach, especially if many variables are studied.

Unfortunately there are many studies for which *no* hypothesis or objective can be determined in the resulting publication. Consequently there is no way to judge whether the study or its conclusions are valid. Alternatively, an objective is stated, the study design tests something else, yet the investigators imply that the conclusions can be applied to the original hypothesis.

Finally, if the hypothesis is not clear the investigator may come to the end of the study and find that crucial data were not collected to answer the question in which he/she was truly interested.

2. EXPERIMENTAL DESIGN

(a) The target population

To which population are results of studies on the group of patients meant to apply? Bias is the term used to describe differences between the target population and the sample on which data for the study were collected. It is obvious that results on heroin users may not be applicable to cocaine users. It may be less obvious that results on a sample of women volunteering for study may not be representative of those not appearing in centers. Detailed description of the study population (that sampled) permits readers to decide if results are applicable to their patients.

(b) Type of study

After determination of the hypothesis or objective, the type of study to answer that question can be selected (Table 11.2). True experiments usually are ethically limited to nonhuman studies.

Descriptive studies

Not all investigations need to be phrased in terms of a testable hypothesis. Some studies may be descriptive only, perhaps to estimate parameters and generate hypotheses for future study designs (exploratory rather than analytic). The extent of growth retardation might be estimated in infants of methadone-treated mothers to determine how many of them, and of infants of drug-free mothers, must be studied to find out if growth retardation is significantly more frequent if mothers use methadone. Conclusions about differences between groups, effects of treatments, or associations with risk factors should not be made from such studies.

119

Table 11.2 Types of studies

Type	Salient features and limitations	Nature of conclusions
Experiment	Study effects of two or more treatments, risk factors. Variables affecting outcomes can be manipulated. Possible with nonhuman subjects.	Manipulation of a factor affects outcome (response) variable
Clinical trial	Equivalent groups of patients concurrently and similarly treated, randomly assigned to comparison groups, e.g. treatment vs. placebo, blindly evaluated.	Differences of patients with regard to outcome variable are due to treatment or protocol
Retrospective survey (case–control)	Observation, not manipulation. Cases selected on abnormal outcome variables and compared with normal outcomes. Cannot provide direct risk estimates. Preferred when outcome is rare.	If cases have a higher frequency of potential risk factor(s) than controls, there is a possible association.
Prospective survey (cohort)	Observation, not manipulation. Cases selected on 'risk' variable(s) and compared to outcomes of controls who are not exposed to 'risk' variable. Can provide risk estimates. Preferred when risk factor is rare.	Higher frequency of poor outcomes in cases (exposed) than in controls (non-exposed) is suggestive of cause and effect
Cross-sectional	Both risk factors and outcome variable are determined simultaneously.	If groups with abnormal outcomes also have higher frequency of potential risk variable, suggestive of associations. Cannot determine whether outcome preceded 'exposure' or vice-versa

Surveys

Particularly in the early history of a field, there may be a need for good descriptive studies from which hypotheses can be generated and subsequently formally tested. The history of the discovery of the infamous association between DES exposure *in utero* and development of vaginal adenocarcinoma began when Scully and Herbst noticed an unusual number of cases of what was previously a rare cancer. This observation stimulated a retrospective (case–control) study in which records of abnormal cases were compared to those of normal controls, in order to search for possible etiologic factors. In this study the suspicious factor turned out to be *in utero* DES exposure of females with cancer. The finale of this line of investigation was a *prospective* study in which selection of the study population was by the proposed risk factor, DES use in pregnancy. All possible outcomes, including vaginal adenocarcinoma, were compared to that in comparable non-exposed populations.

Another example of this same progression of scientific investigations was the *observation* in Australia of an unusual number of cases of a form of congenital cataract in newborns. This was followed by a *retrospective study* which ferreted out rubella infection during pregnancy as a possible etiologic factor. As in the DES story, causation was more firmly established with a *prospective study* of exposed vs. non-exposed mothers.

In summary, descriptive studies are important, but must be defined as such, and conclusions must not be made from them. These studies should then be followed by those in which cases are selected because of an abnormal outcome, controls being selected from those without the abnormal outcome. Both groups' histories are examined for differences to ascertain potential risk factors. Finally, a prospective study is done. The recent observation of birth of an infant with prune belly syndrome to a cocaine user[2] might be pursued by a retrospective study, but this is a rare condition so data may be hard to obtain.

The advantages of a retrospective compared to a prospective study are that the former requires a smaller sample size than the latter and, because the outcomes have already occurred, a retrospective study is cheaper and quicker to conduct. The DES–vaginal adenocarcinoma association was uncovered with only eight cases, each with four controls. The major disadvantages of retrospective studies are that they cannot provide direct risk estimates and can only evaluate the specified outcome. Only a prospective study can hope to answer such patient questions as: 'What is the chance of having a stillbirth if I am using heroin?' One disadvantage of prospective studies is that large numbers are needed in the samples because most patients followed will have normal outcomes so this is an expensive and time-consuming approach. Most studies of the effects of drug abuse on pregnancy are *prospective* because most investigators in this area will have access to patients on drugs. Unfortunately, sample sizes may be small (see Section 4). When the risk factor is rare, case–control studies may not include enough persons who were exposed, to detect a real association. This might be a problem for certain drug studies if drug use is rare. However, retrospective studies may have other useful formats, e.g. dividing women on methadone by whether pregnancy outcome was normal or abnormal might elucidate risk factors within this group.

In pregnancy outcome case–control studies, histories of women having stillbirths might be compared to those with normal liveborn deliveries. Differences between the two groups might include previous pregnancy outcomes, maternal health, and drug use. If any of these are already known to be associated with stillbirths, e.g. maternal health, the sample can be subdivided by that factor and comparisons of drug use made within those groups. If drug use seems to be higher in the group of women having stillbirths even after corrections for other factors affecting pregnancy outcome, then a prospective study should be conducted.

Women using drugs should be compared to women who are drug-free, and one of the outcome variables compared should be frequency of stillbirths. If there is a higher frequency among drug users, that would be suggestive of cause and effect.

A *cross-sectional study* would select a group of women and look both at potential risk and outcome variable frequencies, e.g. pregnancy outcome and frequency of drug use in a sample of women. This type of study can only suggest associations. It will not be clear which of the variables found to be associated temporally preceded the other, so cause and effect cannot be established.

Clinical trials

The *clinical trial* is the design used to assess the effects of therapies, medications, or experimental protocols. Whether paregoric and phenobarbital differ in alleviating specific symptoms of infant withdrawal would be determined by a clinical trial in which equivalent groups of subjects were treated concurrently in two ways. Subjects must be *ramdomly* allocated to the groups. If decisions on which drugs or protocols are to be administered to an individual are made by the physician and/or patient, the reasons for the decision could affect the outcome being studied. Differences observed between those treated with paregoric vs. phenobarbital could not be attributed to the treatment *per se* if not randomly allocated, because they might be explainable by inherent differences of the groups. Randomization can be achieved by assigning a random number obtained from a table or generated by a computer. Randomization tends to allocate unknown factors which affect the response variable between the two groups, so that outcome differences are more likely to be attributable to the treatments, not to inherent differences between the groups. In a publication the *method* of randomization must be described.

In drug abuse studies it may not always be ethical to randomize. Can methadone be withheld even with consent? On the other hand, if the effects of methadone on pregnancy outcome are not established, methadone could be beneficial *or* harmful, therefore is it ethical *not* to conduct a randomized clinical trial? The major problem with just comparing groups that exist, e.g drug-free women with those on methadone, is that other factors relevant to the outcome of interest may differ among the two groups. Those in clinics may be more motivated to care for themselves prenatally. Those on drugs may have poorer nutritional habits. The fact that it is very difficult to achieve comparability for factors other than drug use should not deter investigators from strengthening their conclusions by creative approaches to the problem.

If the patients are infants, it would not be necessary to worry about 'blindness' on the part of the patient; however, adult patients and investigators should be blinded, in particular when subjective evaluations are being made as part of the study – otherwise, suspicion will exist that the observers injected bias, albeit unconsciously, into evaluations depending on their feelings and beliefs regarding the relative efficacies of the drugs (or whatever is being tested).

Table 11.3 Evaluation of clinical trials

Possible reasons for observed differences among groups	Explanation assessed or removed by
1. Chance (sampling varition)	1. Statistical test
2. Inherent differences between groups	2. Randomization (matching, stratification, adjustment optional)
3. Differential handling and evaluation of groups	3. Double-blind
4. True differences	4. Assume possible if other explanations (1–3) unlikely, and results are biologically feasible

Table 11.3 summarizes the construction and evaluation of clinical trials.

(c) Type of variables: confounding, risk or treatment, response (outcome)

On which variables do data need to be collected to answer the question(s) posed in the hypothesis or objective? There will be several classes of variables – those which are the responses or outcome of interest (for example, pregnancy result, birthweight, head circumference), those risk or treatment variables being studied, and potential confounding variables such as age, parity, major maternal illnesses which may also affect response outcomes. The type of variable(s) will ultimately determine choice of statistical analysis, e.g. *t*-tests and correlation coefficients are appropriate for continuous variables (blood pressure, birthweight); chi-square analysis is used for measurement variables which are discrete (boy vs. girl) and for some qualitative variables (nominal classes, e.g. caucasian, black, oriental; ordinal, e.g. ratings on behavioral scales). Non-parametric statistics may be useful for analysis of variables for which assumptions of parametric tests are not met.

Reliability, validity and reproducibility of the data must be assessed. Can different sources of data be used to check reliability? e.g. can urine testing be used to check if mothers are drug-free or are on multiple drugs? Questionnaires have been developed by many groups with reliability checks incorporated into their structure, e.g. by asking for the same information in different ways[3].

Data collection formats must be carefully constructed to elicit all relevant data in an unbiased fashion. The definition of variables, methods of measuring or assessing them, error checks, must be precisely set out *before* the study begins. If clinical classifications are to be made, the rules must be unambiguous and all-inclusive. Patients included in the study cannot be excluded after data are collected, although reasons may be presented for analyzing certain groups separately.

In studies of the effects of drugs, one of the most difficult problems to overcome is that of confounding variables. The biologic outcome variables, e.g. frequency of prematurity, may be affected by nutritional factors, previous pregnancy history and maternal health. The frequencies of congenital malformations are known to vary according to maternal age, race, geographic location and maternal health. If these confounding variables are ignored, their presence may cause increases in abnormal pregnancy outcomes which are spuriously attributed to drug use simply because these high-risk women *also* were more likely to use drugs (see example in Table 11.4). Conversely, improper consideration of these variables could obscure a drug effect if, for example, the 'control' or 'normal' values are spuriously high due to the presence of factors increasing abnormal outcomes. There are several ways to correct for confounding variables: matching, stratification and adjustment. Randomization will tend to equalize confounding factors if samples are large, so these corrective measures are not always necessary.

Table 11.4 Hypothetical data: effect of confounding factors
(a) Outcomes classified by methadone use only

	Methadone	No methadone	Total
Stillborn	10	20	30
Liveborn	40	30	70
	50	50	100
Stillborn frequency	.2	.4	

Conclusion: Methadone may be protective

(b) Outcomes also classified by another variable affecting stillbirths

	Low-risk stillbirth		Total	High-risk stillbirth		Total
	Methadone	No methadone		methadone	No methadone	
Stillborn	4	2	6	6	18	24
Liveborn	36	18	54	4	12	16
	40	20	60	10	30	40
			50	50		
Stillborn frequency	0.1	0.1		0.6	0.6	

Conclusion: *No* effect of methadone on stillbirth frequency

Matching of controls (or of different classes of drug users) is one approach to remove effects of major confounding variables. Random selection of controls from a comparable population is *not* matching. This term refers to deliberate selection of cases because of factors similar to that of a particular case. Care must be taken not to try to match on so many variables that matching is not feasible. It should also be remembered that matched variables cannot be analyzed as risk factors because the patients were selected for these. The frequency of occurrence is controlled by the investigator. Close matching achieves better comparability, but may be difficult to achieve in practice. Usually some tolerance is acceptable, e.g. ages might be required to match within 2 years. Matches can be paired (one on one) or multiple (several controls for each pair). Several control groups may be needed for various comparisons because one control group may not correct for all confounders. Matching should be viewed neither as essential nor as reliably solving the problem of the impact of confounding variables. Demonstrating that mean value of a quantitative trait is the same in matched groups does not assure an unbiased comparison, e.g. complex, nonlinear relationships may exist. Further discussion of complexities of matching may be found in Anderson *et al.*[4].

Stratification means to select cases and controls within categories of a potential confounding variable, e.g. primiparous vs. multiparous. In a clinical trial, randomization of treatments can then be done within each stratum. Special statistical techniques are available for analysis of stratified data.

Another little-used method which is appropriate for drug studies to correct for confounding variables is adjustment by standardization or multivariate (covariate) techniques. In standardization, estimates of outcome variables are made as if the groups being compared were indeed similar with regard to confounding variables. With multivariate techniques, adjustment of the outcome variables is made based on values of confounding variables for each patient. These are reasonable, sometimes preferable alternatives to matching.

(d) Sample size: too small to detect an effect?

This is probably one of the most serious problems facing research to evaluate effects and treatments of drug abuse. Too much emphasis may be placed on negative (non-significant) results when in fact the sample size may have been too small to detect a clinically interesting effect. Freiman *et al.*[5] found that 50/71 medical studies reviewed that reported no treatment effects, had greater than a 10% chance of missing a true improvement over controls as large as 50%. Before beginning a study an estimate should be made of the numbers of patients and controls likely to be recruited. If the sample size is too small to pick up a clinically relevant difference, it may be viewed as a descriptive or a pilot study to be followed with a larger, more definitive study. False reassurance of no effects should not be made. The choice of study design may depend on the realistic estimate of the number of patients available. Centers may pool data (although some analytic problems may arise due to heterogeneity among centers), or the study may be extended for several years to achieve a reasonable sample size. The smaller the real effect, the larger the sample needed to detect it. Conversely, large samples may yield 'statistically significant,' yet biologically useless, results because the effects are real, but very small. To estimate the sample size needed to pick up a specific level of effect, the investigator needs to know:

1. α, the significance level desired, usually 5% or 1%;
2. β, the tolerance error of not detecting the alternative hypothesis that there *is* an effect or association (usually β is 10% or 20%); a related term, the *power,* is the chance of detecting the alternative hypothesis if it is true (power $= 1-\beta$, usually 80-90%);
3. the magnitude of biologic effect or association that would be clinically relevant;
4. the inherent variability of the data.

This information should be published with results of each study so the reader can assess the strength of the conclusions.

(e) Data collection, sample selection

To avoid bias, chance should direct selection of cases, and controls. This can be achieved by simple random sampling in which each patient or control has the same chance of being selected. For both cases and controls the chance of being selected must be unrelated to the potential risk factor. Complex sampling procedures are discussed in Cochran[6].

The source of patients and controls must be considered. Studies of patients from special clinics may show wide variability because of small samples and differing referrral and patient entry criteria. This may account for lack of consistency from results of similar investigations at different clinics. It also means that results of a special clinic may not be extrapolated to a general group of such patients. Population-based studies, although difficult to implement, should be considered before final decisions are made regarding patient care or public policy.

As previously discussed, inclusion and exclusion criteria must be unambiguous. Data collection formats should be tested for clarity, completeness, ease of use and reliability before the study. Procedures for randomization and blinding must be specified.

With regard to data collecting, observer variability can be large enough to obscure biologic results, or to create spurious ones. This is of greater concern the more subjective the evaluations, such as psychological examinations. Blinding the observers regarding source of the subject (control vs. experimental) guards against weighing results according to the observer's biases. This can particularly affect classification of 'doubtful' or 'borderline' outcomes. Bias is usually unconscious rather than deliberate, but in any case the credibility of the study will suffer if blindness is not documented. Subjects of various groups should all be studied by the same observers, or randomized among them. In the analysis, differences among observers should be assessed and corrected for as necessary. Comparisons may be made within each observer's evaluations. If one observer or group of observers evaluates controls, and another the experimental group(s), observer bias is confounded with true group differences. Even with standard tests and measurements, this can be a problem. Only with unassailable end points such as 'dead vs. alive' is this probably not a concern.

Investigators may inflate the strength of their conclusions by mentioning large numbers in publications which present a false impression. The study group may be initially described as 500 women, but when the results of those completing the study are presented, it may only be 30! These papers should be examined with care to determine why women were excluded and how many were lost to follow-up. Attempts should be made to determine who left the study and why, to try to determine the nature of the resulting bias. Perhaps the worse addicts, hence those potentially at highest risk, left. Were abnormal outcomes more likely to be lost to follow-up? There are statistical methods such as life table and survival analysis which may be considered in some studies for censored data (e.g. different lengths of follow-up for each patient). Analysis cannot simply be restricted to those completing the study, or for which all variables are recorded, ignoring patients who change treatments in the midst of the study, or stop complying with the protocol at different points after the study inception, without risking serious bias in the conclusions. Usually this exclusion will serve to paint a rosier picture than justified because those completing the study are healthier, more compliant, more motivated. Loss in the control group might lead to spurious differences with drug groups if the remaining controls at the end of the study are too 'normal', not representative of a drug-free general population.

(f) Controls

Controls are required for almost all studies which purport to form conclusions rather than to be merely descriptive. Statements such as '60% of infants of opiate-addicted mothers are hyperactive' are meaningless unless the frequency of hyperactivity in infants of drug-free mothers is available for comparison. Some investigators have not even attempted to find controls because 'exact matching' is not possible. Controls need not be matched to be useful. They should be randomly drawn, however, from as similar a population of study subjects as possible. If differences in the study outcome, e.g. infant hyperactivity, are found between infants of control vs. drug-addicted mothers, it is true that factors other than drug use may have caused the differences observed (see Section (c)). However, in the absence of controls, *no* conclusions are valid unless the response is so extreme as to be obvious. If *all* infants of heroin addicts *died* in the neonatal period prior to methadone treatment, and now most live, a statistical analysis might not be needed to prove the virtue of methadone. Rarely are such quantum effects observed in research, however.

Comparison with standard values obtained in large segments of the population (height percentiles, Apgar scores) would be the next best approach if controls were impossible to obtain.

Valid comparisons can also be made among users of different levels of the same drug, or of different drug groups. However, conclusions must not extend beyond these target populations.

Sources of cases for retrospective studies include birth defect registries, birth certificates, hospital records and group practices.

Controls must be selected from the same source as were the cases. Investigators should be alert for well-known biases resulting from controls' motivation for volunteering for studies. There is also a well-known bias of recall among mothers with untoward pregnancy outcomes.

It is essential not only to select appropriate controls, but to follow them to the same extent and to give them the same care and observation as cases. If cases are selected early in pregnancy, controls should be also. Historical controls are usually suspect because their use assumes no changes over time in variables affecting outcome other than the one under study. Comparing pregnancy loss rates among heroin users in the past with those now on methadone and attributing changes to methadone ignores other important changes over time in factors affecting pregnancy loss in general.

3. DATA PRESENTATION

Before proceeding with data analysis the data should be displayed to determine its variability and the general nature of the results. Means (averages), standard deviations (variability of the measurements around the mean), and other relevant descriptive statistics should be calculated for continuous variables. Variables should be plotted or graphed to determine their distribution (relative frequency of each value). If the data are normally distributed, there are certain properties of the normal curve which may be useful, e.g. that 95% of the values should be within plus or minus 2 standard deviations. If distributions are asymmetrical, these relationships may not be assumed. Medians, percentiles and ranges are useful for non-normal data. Moreover, most parametric statistical tests are based on assumptions of normality. If the data are *not* normally distributed, they may sometimes be transformed to normal by use of log, square root, and so forth. An alternative is to use non-parametric statistics which do not assume normal distributions[7], e.g. Spearman's rank correlation coefficient is a non-parametric analogue of the Pearson's correlation coefficient; the latter assumes a bivariate normal distribution.

Labelling of the axes of graphs must be clear and must agree with textual presentations. Histograms must be constructed so that unit areas are equal throughout the graph unless otherwise justified. If variables are *not* continuous, bar graphs rather than histograms are appropriate, and class values should not be connected to imply a continuous distribution. Figure 11.1 presents the impression of changes over time, which would suggest data amenable to regression analysis. The impression of independent samples at each ordinate presented is false because the 'x-axis' indicates separate *trials,* not a sequentially increasing variable value measured on the experimental units.

The nature of the relation between two continuous variables should be estimated initially by inspection of plotted data points before statistical analysis. If the relationship is parabolic, use of a linear correlation or regression may yield a slope of zero (a non-significant result). The authors would incorrectly conclude there is no association between, e.g. length

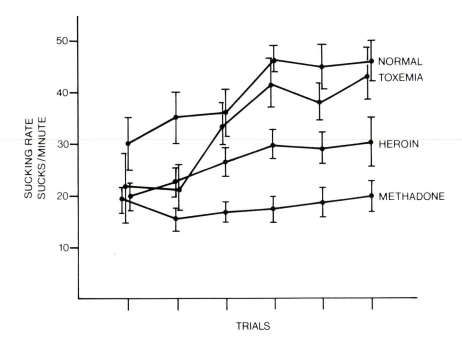

Figure 11.1

of maternal heroin use and infant head circumference, when in fact there is a strong association, but it is not linear. Because a line will always be drawn between data points by a computer program, care must be taken that outliers (perhaps representing data errors or non-representative cases) do not force the slope of a line to be large and significant when there is no real association.

Lack of internal consistency between numbers in the text, tables, and figures, could charitably be attributed to typographic errors. However, poor proof-reading raises doubts about accuracy in the other aspects of data collection and analysis, and confusion as to what results were used for the conclusions. Whether the correct numbers were used in the analysis is also a question when a text says there are 100 mothers of 150 infants, but the table describing characteristics of the sample says there were *150 women*. If a table shows blood pressure of control infants to be 96 (one point in time only) and blood pressures of infants of drug addicts to be 76 and 95 at two points in time, and the conclusion is that blood pressures are elevated by maternal drug use, what figures were compared? If sample sizes differ in various tables, why were units excluded for some analysis?

The sample size in a text was given as 40. Table 11.5 shows the results.

Table 11.5

Age	No. of patients	Postoperative mortality (%)
less than 20 years old	10	10
less than 30 years old	20	18
greater than or equal to 30 years old	20	32
greater than 40 years old	10	40

Adding these patients would yield 60! Inspection reveals the age groups not to be mutually exclusive. Was this to strengthen the authors' conclusion 'postoperative mortality improves steadily with age?'

4. STATISTICAL ANALYSIS

Statistical analyses are required if the conclusion to be sought is that there is a difference among groups, an association between a risk factor and an abnormal outcome, or a change due to a treatment. Because statistical tests are based on certain assumptions, the appropriate one must be chosen to: (a) answer the question stated in the hypothesis or objective; (b) be appropriate for the elements of the experimental design (type of variable, method of selecting the sample) (see Table 11.6). The statistical test is usually phrased in terms of the null hypotheses ('no difference in pregnancy outcomes among women on heroin, on methadone, or drug-free,' 'no association between level of drug use and prematurity,' 'no improvement in drug withdrawal symptoms after treatment with paregoric compared with phenobarbital').

After completing a study the investigator needs to determine whether the results are consistent with the null hypothesis. Are differences among study groups attributable to chance variation or are real differences suggested? To decide this, the data obtained in the study are converted to a test statistic. The distribution of this statistic under the null hypothesis is known. The more unusual the observations if the null hypothesis were true, the larger the value of the test statistic, and the smaller the chance it would occur if the null hypothesis were true. The p-value is the area of the curve enclosing values of the test statistic more extreme than that obtained; this is equivalent to the 'chance' of occurrence of the study results if the null hypothesis were true. Distributions of test statistics are tabulated for easy conversion from test statistics values to p-values. Conceptually, the p-value might be thought of as how many times values (study results) more extreme than that actually obtained would occur by chance alone if the null hypothesis were indeed true and the study were repeated many times. Traditionally, p-values less than 0.01 or less than 0.05 have been designated as 'unusual,' or 'statistically significant.' If the test statistic is in that region, our data lead us to *reject* the null hypothesis. Notice this does not mean the null hypothesis is false. One significant p-value should not be regarded as more than suggestive of a true effect. If a biologic explanation for the effect can be developed, and there is significant deviation from the null hypothesis in other similar studies, the results are more credible.

Table 11.6 Commonly encountered tests of significance

Test	Comments	Varieties	Purpose
t-test	Continuous data	Single sample	Tests on a single sample mean
		Paired	Tests on a sample mean of paired differences
		Two sample (equal variance)	Tests for comparing two independent sample means
Chi-square (χ^2)	Proportions or counted data	Two sample	Tests for comparing two independent proportions
		k sample	Tests for comparing k sample proportions
		Goodness of fit	Tests on k proportions in a single sample
		$r \times c$ contingency	Tests for association
F-test	Continuous data	Analysis of variance	Tests for comparing k sample means
Z-test	Continuous or counted data	Single sample	Tests for a single sample proportion Tests on a single mean when variance known
Correlation	Continuous data, observations in pairs	Pearson product moment	Measure degree of linear association between two variables
Regression	Usually data are continuous; predict one variable from one or several	Simple linear	Tests involving slope of a a line
		Multiple linear	Tests for regression with more than one independent variable regression coefficient

There are several problems which can arise at this stage of the experimental design to invalidate the conclusions of a study.

(a) Inappropriate choice of a statistical test

The choice of a statistical test should be made based on (a) the hypothesis or objective; (b) the type of response and confounding variables; (c) the way the sample was selected for study, including the nature of the controls.

Use of inappropriate tests can have drastic clinical consequences. The t-test is one of the most used and abused statistical methods. It is appropriate to use t-tests to compare means (averages) of quantitative variables in *two* groups. An example would be to compare mean birthweights of infants whose mothers were on methadone maintenance with birthweights of infants whose mothers were drug-free during pregnancy. Glantz[8] reviewed 142 original articles published in one journal and found that 27% used statistical methods incorrectly, and that 44% of all articles that used statistics had errors. Most of the errors were to apply the t-test incorrectly, leading authors of these papers to conclude that 'a treatment produced an effect when the data did not support such a conclusion.' Glantz's review is only one of many similar reviews of articles in the medical literature, all finding depressingly large percentages of papers with invalid conclusions due to faulty study design and/or inappropriate use of statistics. It is sobering to realize that these invalid conclusions are the basis for choice of treatment protocols for patients and for public policy decisions. Major errors in use of a t-test are:

1. *Comparing more than two groups.* If there are more than two groups, the *analysis of variance* method should be used. Recall the definition of a 'p-value.' If the null hypothesis is true, and a 5% significance level is selected, 5/100 experiments will erroneously reject the null hypothesis by obtaining a 'significant' p-value. If there are three groups, and t-tests are computed between groups 1–2, 1–3, and 2–3, the overall p-value will no longer be 5%, but 13%[9]. If a significant difference is found between, for example, controls, methadone users, and heroin users, by Anova, then certain t-tests may be performed among pairs. Guidelines for subsequent use of t-tests after analysis of variance may be found in Scheffe[10]. It is prudent to consult a statistician if more than two groups are in the study design because analysis of variance is fairly complex. Merely plugging data into a computer program for analysis for variance will not necessarily regurgitate correct results.

2. *Performing multiple T-tests on variables in the same data set.* The more tests that are done, the more likely at least one will be significant by chance. This error tends to find more effects or associations than are justified. In addition to correction of this problem by use of multivariate analysis, the significance level desired can be divided by the number of tests performed, and *that* level required for 'significance' in the individual comparisons, e.g. if a level of 5% is desired, and three t-tests are done, a p-value less than 0.016 would be required for each individual test to be significant (0.05/3=0.016). This is a conservative correction called the Bonferroni method, and can be used in general for multiple tests.

From this it can be seen that t-tests should not be used to compare points on curves. An investigator may take glucose measurements at 2, 4, 8 and 24 hours postnatally on infants of control mothers and of drug addicts. If comparisons were made using a t-test for all four time points, the significance level would approximate 20% if the 5% levels in the tables are used. Nor is it appropriate to select by inspection where the greatest difference is and do a single t-test at that point. The two curves are actually large numbers of points at every time between birth and 24 hours. The p-value interpretation is how likely it is that the curves differ significantly by chance. Because there are thousands of points on a curve, to pick out the largest point is biasing toward finding a difference. There may also be more sophisticated analysis to handle this type of study, e.g. analysis of variance of replicate measures sampled over time[10]. Comparison of the curves themselves (slope, intercept, shape) can also be approached through regression techniques.

3. Another error in use of the *t*-test is incorrect choice of the formula to compute this statistic. Denominators vary depending on whether the two groups were matched (paired) or independent, where sample sizes are equal or unequal. For the paired *t*-test there must be *one* control matched to each subject. The formula will differ depending on whether means of two groups are being compared or whether an individual subject is being compared to a group mean.

Use of other statistical tests also poses common problems. Computer aid removes the tedium of computing multiple correlation coefficients, *t*-test and so forth, from large numbers of variables collected on the same patients. Before becoming unduly excited about one 'significant' correlation, for example between 'length of a woman's nose and propensity for drug use,' when many correlations were calculated, the following questions need to be answered:

1. Were appropriate corrections made for multiple comparisons?
2. Does the result make biologic sense?
3. Could this association be due to, e.g. both nose length and drug use being related indirectly through a third variable?

A method of computing *partial correlation coefficients* can be helpful to explore this latter possibility.

Analyzing variables in pairwise fashion (e.g. many 2×2 tables with χ^2 analysis) may be helpful to discern the nature of the results. However, interactions are not detected by these simple tabulations and the problems of multiple comparisons arise, in particular if pairs of variables are correlated.

Statistical methods which need to be considered more for use in drug investigations are:

1. *The Mantel–Haenzel test,* which analyzes differences in outcomes between groups after stratification on risk factor levels or confounding variables.
2. *Life table and survival analysis* which can be applied in some situations where patients are lost to follow-up after varying observation times. This type of data is referred to as *censored.*
3. *Relative risks* for cohort studies; this statistic defines chance of an abnormal outcome if the patient is exposed to the risk factor (e.g. drugs, methadone) as compared to the risk of those unexposed. *Odds ratios* give similar predictions from case-control studies.
4. Methods to handle confounding variables or multiple 'risk' variables include *analysis of covariance* when the outcome and confounding variables are numerical and the treatments categorical. *Logit analysis* may be used to study the effects of a combination of potential risk factors on a dichotomous outcome (dead vs. alive). This method is similar to analysis of covariance. Many confounding variables, either categorical or numerical, may be entered. This method may be better

than stratification in certain circumstances. *Log linear analysis* is useful when the risk, outcome and confounding variables are *all* categorical. This method is similar to analysis of variance. A more complete discussion of these methods may be found in Anderson *et al.*[4].

5. *Discriminant analysis* can be used to ascertain what set of variables distinguishes two groups, e.g. infants with RDS from those without RDS.

6. *Factor analysis* can be used to explore groupings of variables which may affect the outcome.

The most commonly used statistical tests assume that the units of observation are independent. Consequently, repeated measurements on the same set of babies, or inclusion of multiple pregnancies of a woman, require special forms of analysis, not simple t-tests or χ^2.

With regard to replicate measurements, is it more impressive to have 100 blood pressure measurements on a single individual, 10 blood pressure measurements on 10 individuals, or 1 blood pressure measurement on each of 100 individuals? Although the first two sets of measurements can provide valuable information on variability of blood pressure within individuals and on measurment errors, only the last 100 *individuals* justify a claim of a sample size of 100. If 150 women deliver 200 infants (some women had more than one pregnancy) the first 150 pregnancy results should be studied. There are *not* 200 independent units analyzable with simple statistical tests.

5. ARE THE CONCLUSIONS OF THE AUTHOR SUPPORTED BY THE RESULTS OF THE DATA ANALYSIS?

Statements that 'no association was found' or that results were 'significant' should be completely disregarded unless it is clear what variables entered into the comparison, whether the appropriate statistical test was used, what its value was, and what p-value was used to define 'significance.' If the authors claim no association between, for example, time in gestation the woman first came to the clinic, and subsequent hyperactivity in her infant, the reader needs to know if there was enough variability to make such a statement. If all women come in the third month there would be no variability on one of the variables, and no association could be detected even if there would be one in general. If the data were categorical (three levels of drug use), yet the analysis was to compute a correlation coefficient which is appropriate for continuous, quantitative measures, the calculation would not be valid.

Both clinical and statistical 'significance' must be considered. A correlation of 0.2 may be statistically significant but clinically unexciting because a correlation of 0.2 only explains 0.04 (r^2) of the variability in the outcome variable.

Are the conclusions of the author supported by *any* data? A statement such as 'Stillbirth frequencies appear to be related to inadequate prenatal care' cannot be made when nowhere in the paper can data on prenatal care be found, and no mention is made of the measure of this variable or how it was determined to be related to stillbirths.

Conclusions cannot be made that drug use is more prevalent in one ethnic group because the percentage of that ethnic group is higher among pregnant drug clinic patients than in the general population. The correct comparison must be with the percentage of that ethnic group admitted to the routine obstetrical clinic in that hospital (drug-free mothers).

In summary, it is important not to accept conclusions of the author without determining if they are justified by the experimental design, by inspecting tables and graphs presenting results, and by independent assessment of the appropriateness of the analysis and the likelihood the effect (or lack of it) is not due to chance rather than biology. Particularly suspect are papers with several pages of discussion–conclusions yet vague or scant data on which the conclusions are based. Such speculations should be in editorial, not scientific, publications.

REFERENCES

1. Bailar, J. C. III, Louis, T. A., Lavori, P. W. and Polansky, M. (1984). Statistics in practice. Studies without internal controls. *N. Engl. J. Med.*, **311**, 156 – 62
2. Chasnoff, I. J., Burns, W. J., Schnoll, S. H. and Burns, K. A. (1985). Cocaine use in pregnancy. *N. Engl. J. Med.*, **313**, 666 – 9
3. Bennett, A. E. and Ritchie, E. K. (1975). *Questionnaires in Medicine – A Guide to their Design and Use.* (London: Oxford University Press)
4. Anderson, S., Aquier, A., Hauck, W. W., Oakes, D., Vandaele, W. and Weisberg, H. I. (1980). *Statistical Methods for Comparative Studies: Techniques for Bias Reduction.* (New York: John Wiley)
5. Freiman, J. A., Chalmers, T. C., Smith, H. and Kuebler, R. R. (1978). The importance of beta, the type II error and sample size in the design and interpretation of the randomized control trial. *N. Engl. J. Med.* **301**, 682 – 6
6. Cochran, W. G. (1977). *Sampling Techniques.* (New York: Wiley)
7. Siegal, S. (1956). *Non-parametric Statistics for the Behavioral Sciences.* (New York: McGraw-Hill)
8. Glantz, S. A. (1980). Biostatistics: how to detect, correct and prevent errors in the medical literature. *Circulation,* **61**, 1 – 7
9. Zar, J. H. (1974). *Biostatistical Analysis.* (Englewood Cliffs, NJ: Prentice Hall)
10. Scheffe, H. (1959). *The Analysis of Variance.* (New York: John Wiley)

12
Immunologic Function and AIDS in Drug-exposed Infants

KENNETH C. RICH

Drug abuse is associated with a variety of infectious complications. In adults many of these complications are attributable to the use of contaminated materials, the lack of sterile technique for administering intravenous drugs and possibly to the drugs themselves. Other complications are the result of the abnormal lifestyle, such as prostitution, which is required to support the addiction. Infection in infants of drug-addicted mothers is a newly appreciated clinical problem but there is little actual documentation of it in the literature and even less information on the etiology of the susceptibility to infections. This review will examine the information available on the incidence of infections and the possible etiology of the increased risk of infections in drug-abusing patients and their offspring.

INFECTIONS AND IMMUNE FUNCTION IN DRUG ABUSE

Effects of drug abuse on immunologic function

Immune function in human adult opiate abusers ranges from mildly abnormal to severely deficient. Increased concentrations of immuno-globulins in the serum[1], reversed helper to suppressor T-cell ratios[2,3] and increased proportions of null cells[4] have been observed in adult opiate abusers. Many of these abnormalities revert to normal while on methadone maintenance or on discontinuing the opiates[1-4]. Patients with the AIDS-related complex or AIDS have more profound defects (see below).

Experimental animals addicted to morphine have a shorter survival time after infection with *Candida albicans* or *Klebsiella pneumoniae* than non-morphine-treated animals[5]. Furthermore, natural killer activity[6], the number of antibody-producing cells in the circulation[7], and the blasto-genic response to mitogens[8] are reduced in experimental animals receiving morphine. Phagocyte function, including phagocyte count, phagocytic index, killing properties, and superoxide anion production[5] is also reduced. Thus opiates affect *in vitro* immune function as well as overall survival after infection.

A clue to the role of opiates in altering immune function comes from the demonstration that lymphocytes have opiate receptors on the surface. Morphine added to *in vitro* cultures of normal human T-lymphocytes reduces the proportion of total and active T rosettes[9]. The effect is inhibited by the addition of naloxone, an opiate receptor antagonist, suggesting that the T-cells have receptors for morphine[6].

The immunologic consequence of non-opiate drug abuse is variable. Alcohol is commonly abused by drug-addicted mothers. *In vitro* immunologic studies have demonstrated a serum inhibitor of blasto-genesis and chemotaxis in patients with alcoholic cirrhosis[10,11]. Marijuana in large doses suppresses immune function in experimental animals, while in humans, impaired cell-mediated immune function has been reported by some[12] but not all investigators[13].

Infections in infants of drug-abusing mothers

Very little information is available on the incidence of infections in infants of drug-abusing mothers. It has been noted that infants of opiate-abusing mothers have an increased incidence of otitis media during the first year of life compared to infants of non-abusing mothers[14]. We retrospectively examined a population of infants enrolled in the Perinatal Addiction Project of the Northwestern Institute of Psychiatry and the Prentice Women's Hospital and Maternity Center[15]. The infants were divided into those whose mothers abused intravenously administered heroin during pregnancy ($n = 21$) or non-intravenous drugs ($n = 15$), such as phencyclidine or marijuana, and compared them to an age- race and race-matched control population of infants whose mothers did not abuse drugs ($n = 15$). The drug abuse groups were socioeconomically matched. We found that infants of mothers who abused intravenous (i.v.) drugs had an increased incidence of infections compared to those who abused oral drugs or did not abuse drugs (Table 12.1). Persistent oral thrush, bronchiolitis, and chlamydial pneumonia occurred more frequently in offspring of i.v. drug abusers than the oral drug abusers or the normal controls. The thrush was clinically more severe and persistent despite conventional therapy. None of the infants developed severe opportunistic infections or AIDS. Therefore, maternal i.v. drug abuse is associated with an increased incidence of infections for an unknown reason which may or may not be associated with abnormal immune function.

POSSIBLE CAUSES OF INCREASED INFECTIONS IN INFANTS OF DRUG-ABUSING MOTHERS

The cause of the increased infections in infants of drug-abusing mothers is probably multifactoral. The drugs could disrupt the developing immune system or the developing neuroendocrine opioid peptide system. The infants could also acquire a lymphotropic virus at the time of birth. Additionally, extrauterine social factors could play a role. The relative contribution of each of these factors is unknown and will be discussed below.

Table 12.1   Infections in infants of drug-abusing mothers during the first year of life

	Type of drug abuse		
	Intravenous	*Oral*	*None*
Total number of patients	21	15	15
Patients with illness	19	7	8
Number of episodes			
bronchiolitis	9	3	3
Chlamydia pneumonia	3	0	0
thrush	8	1	2
monilia diaper rash	10	1	3
otitis media	10	2	3
Total infectious illnesses	40	7	11

Social factors

The use of illicit drugs by a mother after delivery is disruptive to the social milieu of the infant. It exposes the infant to chaotic social conditions including neglect[16] and maternal alcohol abuse[17]. It increases the risk of inadequate nutrition and of exposure to infectious agents. Protein calorie malnutrition is known to be associated with increased infections and abnormal immune function including depressed macrophage and T-cell function and increased immunoglobulins[18]. However, it is unclear whether the malnutrition is of sufficient magnitude to cause the observed incidence of infections in most infants. Increased exposure to infectious agents results in increased infections and antigen overload, which results in immunologic unresponsiveness[19].

Damage to the developing immune system

The increased infections could be due to damage by drugs to the developing immune system at a critical point in organogenesis. Maternal alcohol abuse is associated with a characteristic pattern of anomalies including central nervous system dysfunction and facial and cardiac anomalies which are the characteristic findings of the fetal alcohol syndrome. The immunologic consequences include a striking increase in the incidence of serious infections and T-cell abnormalities[20]. The similarity between the fetal alcohol syndrome and the congenital diGeorge syndrome (thymic hypoplasia, hypoparathyroidism, and facial and cardiac abnormalities) has been pointed out[21]. A similar syndrome that includes immune abnormalities in infants of mothers abusing other drugs has not been described.

Role of endogenous opioids on immune function

The increased infections in infants of opiate-abusing mothers could also be an effect of damage to the neuroendocrine peptide hormone system at an early point in gestation. The endogenous neuropeptides such as the endorphins and enkephalins have a key role in the body response to stress[22]. They mediate the effect of environmental stress on the immune system probably by binding to lymphocytes and altering immune function. Hypoxic stress[23], advanced labor[24], and neonatal distress[25] all result in enhanced levels of opioids. Foot shock stress in mice is associated with elevated beta-endorphin and enhanced growth of tumors[26]. Whether environmental stress in older infants results in enhanced opioid levels is not known.

Leukocytes have opiate receptors which mediate the effects of opiates on the immune system. Met-enkephalin binds to T-cells[9] and beta-endorphin to lymphoblastoid cells (presumably B-cells)[27] and antibody-producing cells[28]. Opiate receptors are also present on human mono-nuclear phagocytic cells[29] and platelets[30] but few, if any, are present on neutrophils[30]. Naloxone, an opiate antagonist, inhibits binding of opioids to leukocytes under most experimental conditions[28]. Among the activities enhanced by opioids are spontaneous cytotoxicity in man[31], lymphocyte proliferative response in rats[32], and mononuclear cell chemotaxis in man[33]. The suppressed functions include the generation of a T-cell-dependent chemotactic factor for lymphocyte chemotaxis which is mediated through PGE_2[34], the blastogenic response to mitogens in man[35] and antibody formation in mice[36].

Exogenous opiates may affect the ability of the endogenous opioids to respond to stress. In animal preparations, occupation of opiate receptors in the central nervous system by morphine may trigger a negative feedback mechanism which leads to reduced biosynthesis or release of opioid peptides[37]. In mice, prolonged morphine administration does not change met-enkephalin levels or opiate receptor density in the brain, although receptor density is increased with chronic naloxone administration[38]. Neonatal morphine causes long-lasting changes (greater than 6 months) in forebrain opiate receptors in mice[39]. It is not known whether a similar long-lasting change occurs in the immune system opioid receptors and the receptor-mediated function, although it is an attractive possibility. These studies show that there is a modulation of the immune function by the endogenous opioids and that the endogenous system in turn is affected by exogenous opiates.

Lymphotropic virus infection

Adult i.v. drug abuse patients frequently become infected with lymphotropic viruses. Infection with HTLV-III results in AIDS or the AIDS-related complex (described below). Cytomegalovirus (CMV) and Epstein–Barr virus (EBV) infections are common and have adverse effects on the immune system. For example, both acute and chronic EBV infection alter T-cell function[40,41]. In experimental animals CMV suppresses the expression of the primary humoral and cellular immune responses[42]. Thus viral infection of the infant via the mother could result in immune dysfunction, although it does not cause lasting dysfunction in a majority of patients.

In summary, a number of events may potentially cause immune dysfunction in infants of drug-addicted mothers. However, the data are insufficient at present to determine the etiology in most cases.

ACQUIRED IMMUNE DEFICIENCY SYNDROME (AIDS) IN INFANTS

AIDS is a disorder characterized by increased susceptibility to opportunistic infections in previously healthy hosts. It is very closely related to infection with HTLV-III, a retrovirus which affects T-lymphocytes and causes a profound immune defect in some but not all patients infected with the virus[43]. The spread in a community is determined by social factors since the virus is transmitted by blood and some body fluids[44]. About 60% of heterosexual adults with AIDS have a history of abuse of i.v. drugs[45]. The majority of infants with AIDS are offspring of i.v. drug abusers[46] but offspring of Haitians[47] and infants infected by virus containing blood have been reported[48]. The precise mechanism of spread of the virus between mother and infant in the case of an infected mother is not clear, but it is likely that it occurs through the maternal/fetal admixture of blood at the time of delivery.

Clinical presentation of AIDS in infants

The original report of AIDS in an infant was of an infant who developed hepatosplenomegaly, generalized lymphadenopathy and immune deficiency after receiving a blood transfusion from an adult who later developed AIDS[48]. In the three largest series of infants, most of the mothers were either asymptomatic and in a group known to be at increased risk of developing AIDS (prostitutes, i.v. drug abusers, or Haitians) or actually had AIDS[46,47,49]. In the study by Rubenstein et al.[49] seven patients ranging in age from 11 months to 5 years were found to have generalized adenopathy, hepatosplenomegaly and diffuse interstitial pneumonia. The mothers of five were either i.v. drug abusers or sexually promiscuous. Oleske et al.[46] reported on eight children who had an otherwise unexplained immunodeficiency with depressed cell-mediated immunity, hypergammaglobulinemia, and recurrent febrile illnesses. Four of the children died. All had a household exposure to one or more persons with known risk factors for AIDS including seven i.v. drug abusers. A group of infants in Florida who were mostly Haitian (12/14) has been reported[47]. Two of the infants were offspring of i.v. drug abusers. Three half-sibling infants of an i.v. drug abuser who did not have clinically apparent AIDS have also been reported[50]. Not all infants born of mothers with AIDS have developed AIDS[51].

The clinical symptoms most frequently seen in AIDS in infants include chronic interstitial pneumonitis, hepatosplenomegaly, and failure to thrive[51]. Persistent thrush, bacterial infections and chronic diarrhea are also common. These symptoms must be distinguished from those due to a congenital immune deficiency.

The AIDS-related complex (ARC) is a milder form of immunodeficiency in which the patient is HTLV-III antibody positive and has a syndrome characterized by lymphadenopathy and thrush[52]. A proportion of ARC patients go on to develop the complete AIDS syndrome. Interpretation of the risk of progression from ARC to AIDS is difficult because of the long incubation period for AIDS which is estimated in adults to be several years[53].

Laboratory findings in AIDS

The prominent immunologic laboratory findings in AIDS include poly-clonal increase in immunoglobulins and reversed T4/T8 (helper/ suppressor) T-cell ratio due to a decrease in the T4 cells[46,47,49]. These findings are not unique to AIDS. The reversal of the T4/T8 ratio is seen in a number of other conditions including following routine tetanus immunization[54]. The patients may also be lymphopenic, deficient in mitogen and antigen stimulation of lymphocytes *in vitro*[46,47,49], have elevated levels of thymic hormones such as alpha-1-thymosin[55], and have circulating immune complexes[49]. Gamma-interferon production is depressed although the ability of lymphocytes to respond to it is generally normal[56] while interleukin-2 (IL-2) or T-cell growth factor production is normal but the number of IL-2 receptors on lymphocytes is depressed[57]. AIDS patients are deficient in antibody production against specific antigens[58]. Overall, these defects result in the inability to respond to some antigens because of a lack of inducer lymphocyte function and result in the repeated infections with opportunistic infections observed in these patients.

An enzyme-linked immunoassay (ELISA) for HTLV-III antibody has recently become available, and is potentially useful for identifying patients at risk for AIDS. However, it is not diagnostic for AIDS. Antibodies are present in about 80% of adult AIDS patients[59] but are also present in a high proportion of patients in high-risk groups who are asymptomatic and, therefore, cannot be diagnosed as having AIDS. For example, 87% of New York i.v. drug abusers have antibodies[60]. Conversely, patients may have HTLV-III in their lymphocytes but have no antibody response to the virus[61]. The more specific but less sensitive antibody test is done by the Western Blot techniques but is generally available only on a research basis[59]. A positive test in an infant must therefore be interpreted with caution, and take into account the possible transplacental passage to the fetus of maternal IgG antibody as well as the observation of the high proportion of asymptomatic antibody-positive individuals.

Prognosis and treatment of AIDS in infants

The prognosis in childhood AIDS is poor, but precise data are difficult to establish. Thirty-five patients who were reported to the Centers for Disease Control and met the criteria for AIDS had a mean age of onset at 5 months, a mean age at diagnosis of opportunistic infection of 12 months and a mean age at death for the 24 who died of 14 months[62]. In adult AIDS, 5–19% of seropositive homosexual men develop AIDS within 2 - 5 years after they are known to be serology positive while an additional 25% develop ARC[53]. The ultimate prognosis is not known.

Treatment of AIDS has been disappointing. Bone marrow transplantation[63] and treatment with interferon and with IL-2[64] have been attempted without notable success in adults. The difficulty in treatment is due in part to the fact that substantial damage has been done to the immune system by the time the diagnosis is made. Any attempt to engraft new lymphocytes is thwarted by infection of the newly engrafted cells by the virus. Infants diagnosed as having AIDS should receive prophylaxis for *Pneumonocystis carinii* with trimethoprim–sulfamethoxazole, and should receive monthly immune serum globulin since antibody function is poor.

It is necessary to take some precautions to prevent the spread of the HTLV-III virus in infants among contacts. It is known that the virus may be transmitted by infected persons to their heterosexual partners[65]. Furthermore, the virus has been isolated from numerous secretions including saliva[66]. Infection control guidelines for adult AIDS patients have been published[67]. The risk of spread within households by means other than sexual contact appears to be small. In a small study of infected infants cared for by foster parents, no seroconversion by ELISA assay was observed. Furthermore, two of three siblings of AIDS patients did not convert despite living in the same household[68]. However, further studies are needed to determine the extent of conversion within families and the risks to other household members. In the meantime it would be prudent to not allow the sharing of toys and pacifiers contaminated with secretions. In addition, behavior considered 'normal' in a small child, such as biting, also carries a risk for spread. Other precautions are generally those used to prevent spread of hepatitis.

SUMMARY

Infants of intravenous drug-abusing mothers have an increased incidence of infections. The etiology of increased incidence is unclear at present but a number of possibilities have been raised. Adult drug abusers have significant immune abnormalities, and experimental animals chronically exposed to opiates have shorter survival times after infection. Lymphocytes have opiate receptors which may mediate the effects of opiates on the immune system. Whether this is a direct effect of opiates, or of alterations in the endogenous opioid peptide response to stress or an infection with a lymphotropic virus is unknown and is a major topic of research interest at present.

AIDS is another consequence of maternal drug abuse in the infant. The HTLV-III virus can be transmitted vertically from an infected mother to the infant. In preliminary studies the risk of horizontal transmission from the infant to others in the household appears to be low. Not all patients infected with the virus have developed the clinical syndrome of AIDS in short-term follow-up studies. Symptomatic patients with AIDS show marked deficiencies in T-cell inducer function as well as other immunologic abnormalities, and develop repeated opportunistic infections. Treatment thus far has been disappointing. Therefore, infants of drug-abusing mothers require careful follow-up with full cognizance of the potential spectrum of infectious and immunologic abnormalities that they can exhibit.

REFERENCES

1. Brown, S. M., Stimmel, B., Taub, R. N., Kochwa, S. and Rosenfield, R. E. (1974). Immunologic dysfunction in heroin addicts. *Arch. Intern. Med.,* **134,** 1001 – 6
2. Layon, J., Idris, A., Warzynski, M., Sherer, R., Brauner, D., Patch, O., McCulley, D. and Orris, P. (1984). Altered T-lymphocyte subsets in hospitalized intravenous drug abusers. *Arch. Intern. Med.,* **144,** 1376 – 80
3. Mol, B., Emeson, E. E. and Small, C. (1982). Inverted ratio of inducer to suppressor T-lymphocyte subsets in drug abusers with opportunistic infections. *Clin. Immunol. Immunopathol.,* **25,** 417 – 23
4. McDonough, R. J., Madden, J. J., Falek, A., Shafer, D. A., Pline, M., Gordon, D., Bokos, P., Kuehnle, J. C. and Mendelson, J. (1980). Alteration of T and null lymphocyte frequencies in the peripheral blood of human opiate addicts: in vivo evidence for opiate receptor sites on T lymphocytes. *J. Immunol.,* **125,** 2539 – 43
5. Tubaro, E., Borelli, G., Croce, C., Cavallo, G. and Santiangeli, C. (1983). Effect of morphine on resistance to infection. *J. Infect. Dis.,* **148,** 656 – 66
6. Shavit, Y., Lewis, J. W., Terman, G. W., Gale, R. P. and Liebeskind, J. C. (1984). Opioid peptides mediate the suppressive effect of stress on natural killer cell cytotoxity. *Science,* **223,** 188 – 90
7. Gungor, M., Genc, E., Sagduyu, H. and Koyuncuoglu, H. (1980). Effect of chronic administration of morphine on primary immune response in mice. *Experimentia,* **36,** 1309 – 10
8. Law, J. S., Watanabe, K. and West, W. L. (1978). Morphine effects on the responsiveness of lymphocytes to Concanavalin A. *Pharmacologist,* **20,** 231 (abstr.)
9. Wybran, J., Appelboom, T., Famaey, J. P. and Govaerts, A. (1979). Suggestive evidence for receptors for morphine and methionine-enkephalin on normal human blood T lymphocytes. *J. Immunol.* **124,** 1068 – 70
10. Young, G. P., Dudley, F. J. and Van Der Wenden, M. B. (1979). Suppressive effects of alcoholic liver disease sera on lymphocyte transformation. *Gut,* **20,** 833 – 9
11. Van Epps, D. E., Strickland, R. G. and Williams, R. C. (1975). Inhibitors of leukocyte chemotaxis in alcoholic liver disease. *Am. J. Med.,* **59,** 200 – 7
12. Nahas, G. G., Suciu-Foca, N., Armand, J. P. and Morishima, A. (1974). Inhibition of cellular-mediated immunity in marijuana smokers. *Science,* **183,** 419 – 20
13. Silverstein, M. J. and Lessin, P. J. (1974). Normal skin test response in chronic marijuana users. *Science,* **186,** 740 – 1
14. Rosen, T. S. and Johnson, H. L. (1982). Children of methadone-maintained mothers: follow-up to 18 months of age. *J. Pediatr.,* **101,** 192 – 6
15. Chasnoff, I. J. and Rich, K. C. (1984). Increased infections in infants of opiate-abusing mothers. *Pediatr. Res.,* **18,** 254A
16. Oleske, J. M. (1977). Experiences with 118 infants born to narcotic-using mothers. *Clin. Pediatr.,* **16,** 418 – 23
17. Finnegan, L. P. (1981). The effects of narcotics and alcohol on pregnancy and the newborn. *N.Y. Acad. Sci.,* **362,** 136 – 57
18. Smythe, P. M., Schonland, M., Brereton-Stiles, G. G., Coovadia, H. M., Grace, H. J., Loening, W. E., Mafoyane, A., Parent, M. A. and Vos, G. H. (1971). Thymolymphatic

deficiency and depression of cell mediated immunity in protein calorie malnutrition. *Lancet*, **2**, 939 – 44

19. Bixler, G. S. and Booss, J. (1980). Establishment of immunologic memory concurrent with suppression of the primary immune response during acute cytomegalovirus infection of mice. *J. Immunol.*, **125**, 893 – 6

20. Johnson, S., Knight, R., Marmer, D. J. and Steele, R. W. (1981). Immune deficiency in fetal alcohol syndrome. *Pediatr. Res.*, **15**, 908 – 11

21. Ammann, A. J., Wara, D. W., Cowan, M. J., Barrett, D. J. and Stiehm, R. (1982). The diGeorge syndrome and the fetal alcohol syndrome. *Am. J. Dis. Child.*, **136**, 906 – 8

22. Adar, R. (ed.) (1981). *Psychoneuroimmunology.* (New York: Academic Press).

23. Yanagida, H. and Corssen, G. (1981). Respiratory distress and beta-endorphin-like immunoreactivity in humans. *Anesthesia*, **55**, 515 – 19

24. Goland, R. S., Wardlaw, S. L., Stark, R. I. and Frantz, A. G. (1981). Human plasma B-endorphin during pregnancy, labor, and delivery. *J. Clin. Endocrinol. Metab.*, **52**, 74 – 8

25. Shaaban, M. M., Hung, T. T., Hoffman, D. I., Lobo, R. A. and Goebelsmann, U. (1982). B-Endorphin and B-lipotropin concentrations in umbilical cord blood. *Am. J. Obstet. Gynecol.*, **144**, 560 – 8

26. Lewis, J. W., Shavit, Y., Terman, G. W., Nelson, L. R., Gale, R. P. and Liebeskind, J. C. (1983). Apparent involvement of opioid peptides in stress-induced enhancement of tumor growth. *Peptides*, **4**, 635 – 8

27. Hazum, E., Chang, K. J. and Cuatrecasas, P. (1979). Specific nonopiate receptors for B-endorphin. *Science*, **205**, 1033 – 5

28. Lefkowitz, S. S. and Chiang, C. Y. (1975). Effects of certain abused drugs on hemolysis forming cells. *Life Sci.*, **17**, 1763 – 8

29. Lopker, A., Abood, L. G., Hoss, W. and Lionetti, F. J. (1980). Stereoselective muscarinic acetylcholine and opiate receptors in human phagocytic leukocytes. *Clin. Pharmacol.*, **29**, 1361 – 5

30. Mehrishi, J. N. and Mills, I. H. (1983). Opiate receptors on lymphocytes and platelets in man. *Clin. Immunol. Immunopathol.*, **27**, 240 – 9

31. Matthews, J. I., Froelich, C. J., Sibbitt, W. J. and Bankhurst, A. D. (1983). Enhancement of natural cytotoxicity by B-endorphin. *J. Immunol.*, **130**, 1658 – 62

32. Gilman, S. C., Schwartz, J. M., Milner, R. J., Bloom, F. E. and Feldman, J. D. (1982). B-Endorphin enhances lymphocyte proliferative responses. *Proc. Natl. Acad. Sci.*, **79**, 4226 – 30

33. Van Epps, D. E. and Saland, L. (1984). B-Endorphin and met-enkephalin stimulate human peripheral blood mononuclear cell chemotaxis. *J. Immunol.*, **132**, 3046 – 53

34. Brown, S. L. and Van Epps, D. E. (1985). Suppression of T lymphocyte chemotactic factor production by the opioid peptides B-endorphin and met-enkephalin. *J. Immunol.*, **134**, 3384 – 9

35. McCain, H. W., Lamster, I. B., Bozzone, J. M. and Grbic, J. T. (1982). B-Endorphin modulates human immune activity via non-opiate receptor mechanisms. *Life Sci.*, **13**, 1619 – 24

36. Johnson, H. M., Smith, E. M., Torres, B. A. and Blalock, J. E. (1982). Regulation of the in vitro antibody response by neuroendocrine hormones. *Proc. Natl. Acad. Sci.*, **79**, 4171 – 4

37. Jhamandas, K., Yaksh, T. L. and Go, V. L. (1984). Acute and chronic morphine modifies the in vivo release of methionine enkephalin-like immunoreactivity from the cat spinal cord and brain. *Brain Res.*, **297**, 91 – 103

38. Brunello, N., Volterra, A., Di Giulio, A. M., Cuomo, V. and Racagni, G. (1984). Modulation of opioid system in C57 mice after repeated treatment with morphine and naloxone: biochemical and behavioral correlates. *Life Sci.*, **34**, 1669 – 78

39. Handelmann, G. E. and Quirion, R. (1983). Neonatal exposure to morphine increases mu-opiate binding in the adult. *Eur. J. Pharmacol.*, **94**, 357 – 8

40. Weigle, K. A., Sumaya, C. V. and Montiel, M. M. (1983). Changes in T-lymphocyte subsets during childhood Epstein–Barr virus infectious mononucleosis *J. Clin. Immunol.*, **3**, 151 – 5

41. Kibler, R., Lucas, D. O., Hicks, M. J., Poulos, B. T. and Jones, J. F. (1985). Immune function in chronic active Epstein – Barr virus infection. *J. Clin. Immunol.*, **5**, 46 – 53

42. Bixler, G. S. and Booss, J. (1980). Establishment of immunologic memory concurrent with suppression of the primary immune response during acute cytomegalovirus infection of mice. *J. Immunol.,* **125,** 893 – 6

43. Gallo, R. C., Salahuddin, S. Z., Popovic, M., Shearer, G. M., Kaplan, M., Haynes, B. F., Palker, T. J., Redfield, R., Oleske, J. and Safai, B. (1984). Frequent detection and isolation of cytopathic retroviruses (HTLV-III) from patients with AIDS and at risk for AIDS. *Science,* **225,** 500 – 3

44. Girsch, M. S., Wormser, G. P., Schooley, R. T., Go, D. D., Felsenstein, D., Hopkins, C., Holine, C., Duncanson, F., Sarngadharan, M., Saxinger, C. and Gallo, R. (1985). Risk of nosocomial infection with human T-cell lymphotropic virus III (HTLV-III). *N. Engl. J. Med.,* **312,** 1 – 4

45. CDC (1982). Update on Kaposi's sarcoma and opportunistic infection in previously healthy persons. *MMWR,* **31,** 17

46. Oleske, J., Minnefor, A., Cooper, R., Thomas, K., Cruz, A. D., Ahdieh, H., Guerrero, I., Hoshi, V. V. and Desposito, F. (1983). Immune deficiency syndrome in children. *J. Am. Med. Assoc.,* **249,** 2345 – 9

47. Scott, G. B., Buck, B. E., Letterman, J. G., Bloom, F. L. and Parks, W. P. (1984). Acquired immunodeficiency syndrome in infants. *N. Engl. J. Med.,* **310,** 76 – 81

48. Ammann, A. J., Cowan, M. J., Wara, D. W., Weintrub, P., Dritz, S., Goldman, H. and Perkins, H. A. (1983). Acquired immunodeficiency in an infant: possible transmission by means of blood products. *Lancet,* **1,** 956 – 8

49. Rubinstein, A., Sicklick, M., Gupta, A., Bernstein, L., Klein, N., Rubinstein, E., Spigland, I., Fruchter, L., Litman, N., Lee, H. and Hollander, M. (1983). Acquired immunodeficiency with reversed T4/T8 ratios in infants born to promiscuous and drug-addicted mothers. *J. Am. Med. Assoc.,* **249,** 2350 – 6

50. Cowan, M. J., Hellmann, D., Chudwin, D., Wara, D. W., Chang, R. S., Ammann, A. J. *et al.* (1984). Maternal transmission of acquired immune deficiency syndrome. *Pediatrics.,* **73,** 382 – 6

51. Shannon, K. M. and Ammann, A. (1985). Acquired immune deficiency syndrome in childhood. *J. Pediatr.,* **106,** 332 – 42

52. Centers for Disease Control (1982). Persistent, generalized lymphadenopathy among homosexual males. *MMWR,* **31,** 249 – 51

53. Goedert, J. J., Sarngadharan, M. G., Biggar, R. J., Weiss, S. H., Winn, D. M., Grossman, R. J., Greene, M. H., Bodner, A. J., Mann, D. L., Strong, D. M., Gallo, R. C. and Blattner, W. A. (1984). Determinants of retrovirus (HTLV-III) antibody and immunodeficiency conditions in homosexual men) *Lancet,* **2,** 711 – 16

54. Eibl, M. M., Mannhalter, J. W. and Zlabinger, G. (1984). Abnormal T-lymphocyte subpopulations in healthy subjects after tetanus booster immunization. *N. Engl. J. Med.,* **310,** 198 – 9

55. Lederman, M. M., Ratnoff, O. D., Scillian, J. J., Jones, P. K. and Schacter, B. (1983). Impaired cell-mediated immunity in patients with classic hemophilia. *N. Engl. J. Med.,* **308,** 79 – 83

56. Murray, H. W., Rubin, B. Y., Masur, H. and Roberts, R. B. (1984). Impaired production of lymphokines and immune (gamma) interferon in the acquired immuno-deficiency syndrome. *N. Engl. J. Med.,* **310,** 883 – 9

57. Prince, H. E., Kermani-Arab, V. and Fahey, J. L. (1984). Epressed interleukin 2 receptor expression in acquired immune deficiency and lymphadenopathy syndromes. *J. Immunol.,* **133,** 1313 – 17

58. Lane, H. C., Masur, H., Edgar, L. C., Whalen, G., Rook, A. H. and Fauci, A. S. (1983). Abnormalities of B-cell activation and immunoregulation in patients with the acquired immunodeficiency syndrome. *N. Engl. J. Med.,* **309,** 453 – 8

59. Sarngadharan, M. G., Popovic, M., Bruch, L., Schupbach, F. and Gallo, R. C. (1984). Antibodies reactive with human T-lymphotropic retrovirus (HTLV-III) from patients with AIDS and at risk for AIDS. *Science,* **224,** 500

60. Spira, T. J., Des Jarlais, D. C., Marmor, M., Yancovitz, S., Friedman, S., Garber, J., Cohen, H., Cabradilla, C. and Kalyanaraman, V. C. (1984). Prevalence of antibody to lymphadenopathy-associated virus among drug detoxification patients in New York. *N. Engl. J. Med.,* **311,** 467 – 8

61. Salahuddin, S. Z., Groopman, J. E., Markham, P. D., Sarngadharan, M. G., Redfield R. R., McLane, M. F., Essex, M., Sliski, A. and Gallo, R. C. (1984). HTLV-III in symptom-free seronegative persons. *Lancet,* **2,** 1418 – 20
62. Thomas, P. A., Jaffe, H. W., Spira, T. J., Reiss, R., Guerrero, I. C. and Auerbach, D. (1984). Unexplained immunodeficiency in children. *J. Am. Med. Assoc.,* **252,** 639 – 44
63. Hassett, J. M., Zaroulis, C. G., Greenberg, M. L. and Siegal, F. P. (1982). Bone marrow transplantation in AIDS. *N. Engl. J. Med.,* **309,** 665
64. Lane, H. C., Masur, H., Rook, A., Quinnan, G. V., Gelmann, E., Steis, R., Longo, D., Palestine, A., Machu, A. and Fauci, A. S. (1984). Treatment of patients with acquired immunodeficiency syndrome with interleukin-2 or gamma-interferon (Abstr.) *Clin. Res.,* **32,** 351A
65. Harris, C., Small, C. B., Klein, R. S., Friedland, G. H., Moll, B., Emeson, E. E., Spigland, I. and Steigbigel, N. H. (1983). Immunodeficiency in female sexual partners of men with the acquired immunodeficiency syndrome. *N. Engl. J. Med.,* **308,** 1181 – 4
66. Markham, P. D. (1985). Biologic properties and isolation of HTLV-III, pp. 805 – 7. In Fauci, A. S. (moderator). The acquired immunodeficiency syndrome: an update. *Ann. Intern. Med.,* **102,** 800 – 13
67. Conte, J. E., Hadley, W. K. and Sane, M. (1983). Infection control guidelines for patients with the acquired immunodeficiency syndrome (AIDS). *N. Engl. J. Med.,* **309,** 740
68. Kaplan, J. E., Oleske, J. M., Getchell, J. P. *et al.* (1985). Evidence against transmission of human T-lymphotropic virus/lymphadenopathy-associated virus in families of children with the acquired immunodeficiency syndrome. *Pediatr. Infect. Dis.,* **4,** 468 – 71

13
Legal Issues in Perinatal Addiction

MITCHELL J. WIET

The following considerations are addressed in this treatise:

1. the fundamental conflict between child abuse and neglect reporting laws on the one hand, and patient treatment confidentiality laws on the other;
2. the so-called 'Baby Doe' laws and regulations including the concept of 'medical neglect'; and
3. an investigation of an existing legal infrastructure for non-voluntary perinatal drug addiction treatment.

This monograph concludes with an argument in favor of such non-voluntary treatment.

CHILD ABUSE AND NEGLECT–REPORTING LAWS

It is often erroneously thought that child abuse and neglect reporting laws are exclusively a matter of statutes and administrative regulations enacted by state legislatures and promulgated by state administrative bodies. That simply is not so. In 1974 the federal Child Abuse Prevention and Treatment Act of 1974[1] became law and was significantly amended by the Child Abuse Amendments of 1984[2]. Further, the Code of Federal Regulations sets forth administrative rules for the implementation of these federal laws[3].

The purpose of these federal laws and regulations is to create a federal framework and criteria which the several states must meet by enacting state laws and establishing consistent state regulations as a condition of their receiving and continuing to receive federal funding and support for state programs concerning the enforcement of child abuse and neglect laws, including the reporting requirements under such laws.

Thus, with some minor differences, state child abuse and neglect reporting laws resemble each other in basic content because each state enacting them is attempting to meet the federally established criteria. The

Illinois Abused and Neglected Child Reporting Act[4] is used as a model of such state laws throughout this writing and is hereinafter referred to as the 'Illinois Act.'

Typically, these state laws will charge a specific state agency with enforcement responsibility, will establish key definitions of child abuse and child neglect, will specify persons with reporting responsibilities, will provide for specified persons taking temporary protective custody of a suspected abused child and will provide for immunity from civil and criminal liability as the result of reporting child abuse or neglect cases[5]. The state, and not the federal government, has direct enforcement responsibility.

While it is clear that the child abuse reporting laws apply to neonates born alive, a threshold legal question is whether these laws have prenatal application. In *Reyes* v. *Superior Court*[6], a California Appellate Court held that a fetus was not a 'child' for purposes of supporting a felony child endangering charge against an addicted expectant mother. Also, in *Matter of Dittrick Infant*[7], the Michigan Court of Appeals held that the state code did not apply to the unborn in circumstances not involving prenatal addiction.

However, more recently, the Michigan Appellate Court has held in *In the Matter of Baby X*[8] that prenatal maternal drug addiction is sufficient to establish the court's jurisdiction under Michigan neglected child laws where the petition for temporary custody was filed by the state after the birth of the child. Further, in cases not clearly involving prenatal drug addiction, courts are now increasingly using the child abuse reporting laws and/or *parens patriae*[9] theory to extend court jurisdiction to protect the unborn fetus. Decisions in New Jersey[10], Georgia[11], Colorado[12] and Illinois[13] support holdings requiring expectant mothers to undergo Caesarean sections and/or blood transfusions in order to protect fetal life through live birth against their express wishes on religious and other grounds.

Thus, the law is evolving toward extending jurisdiction under the child abuse and neglect reporting laws to the unborn viable fetus. While the legal duty to report such instances is not yet clear, health care professionals would have the benefit of statutory immunity when they, as a matter of professional judgement, report such prenatal instances. Of course, the reporting of an instance of prenatal addiction can always be based on a concern for the abuse or neglect of older siblings in the same household.

On its face, the Illinois Act contains language of mandate for the immediate reporting of child abuse and neglect and specifically places the reporting obligation on a broad range of health care professionals including physicians, surgeons, nurses, hospital administrators, social workers and registered psychologists[14]. The reporting standard is 'reasonable cause to believe'[14] that a child is abused or neglected, not metaphysical certainty. Per an Opinion Letter of the Illinois Attorney General, 'reasonable cause to believe' means 'known or suspected' as per the Code of Federal Regulations, Title 45, §1340.3–3(d) (2)[15]. Willful failure to report can be a grounds for professional licensure suspension or revocation. In Illinois this is true for physicians, nurses, podiatrists, psychologists, dentists and social workers[16].

The Illinois Act, as similar laws in most states, provides for temporary protective custody of a child suspected of being abused or neglected[17]. It is not mandatory, but discretionary. It is invocable only by a physician treating the child, by a local law enforcement officer or by an employee of the Department of Children and Family Services (DCFS). In order to be invoked, three elements must be simultaneously extant:

1. reason to believe the existence of 'imminent danger' to the child's life or health;
2. the person responsible is unavailable or has been asked for and refuses temporary custody; and
3. there is no time to apply for a court order in order to avert the 'imminent danger' to the child's life or health.

Temporary custody may be used by the physician to give emergency medical treatment to a child. DCFS is to be notified promptly after temporary custody is invoked as well as the hospital administrator who then becomes responsible for the further care of the child.

Most states provide for immunity from criminal and civil liability for reporting abuse and neglect cases and for the taking of temporary custody. The Illinois Act so provides and sets forth a statutory presumption of having acted in good faith[18].

CONFIDENTIALITY LAWS – DRUG ABUSE PATIENT TREATMENT RECORDS

Outside of certain narrow exceptions, the federal Drug Abuse Office and Treatment Act of 1972[19] and the implementing administrative rules set forth in the Code of Federal Regulations[20], purport to confer absolute and blanket confidentiality protection on patient treatment records for drug abuse treatment in such federally assisted programs. Indeed, section 408(a) of the 1972 Act[21] provides:

Records of the identity, diagnosis, prognosis, or treatment of any patient which are maintained in connection with the performance of any drug abuse prevention function conducted, regulated, or directly or indirectly assisted by any department or agency of the United States shall, except as provided in subsection (c), be confidential and be disclosed only for the purposes and under the circumstances expressly authorized under subsection (b) of this section.

The 1972 Act permits disclosure of such records only pursuant to specific patient written consent[22], or, without consent, to medical personnel to the extent necessary to meet a bona fide medical emergency[23], or for the purpose of conducting program scientific and financial audits[24], or upon court order after application showing good cause therefor[25]. Wrongful disclosures are punishable by fines of from $500 to $5000[26]. Thus, except for these very narrow circumstances, these federal laws would prohibit disclosure of treatment information concerning an addicted mother for purposes of child abuse or neglect reporting[27].

Some state laws also purport to proscribe disclosure of drug addiction treatment patient information. Examples are mental health codes and the physician–patient privilege. In Illinois these confidentiality protections are respectively codified under the Mental Health and Developmental Disabilities Confidentiality Act[28] and under the Illinois Code of Civil Procedure[29].

PREDOMINANCE OF CHILD ABUSE AND NEGLECT REPORTING LAWS

The conflict between child abuse reporting laws and confidentiality laws is often mischaracterized as a conflict between state and federal laws only. Such misconceptions lose sight of the fact that state mandatory child abuse and neglect reporting is a requirement of the federal Child Abuse Prevention and Treatment Act of 1974[1] mentioned above. The real conflict, then, is a conflict between federal laws at the root, i.e. between the Child Abuse Prevention and Treatment Act of 1974[1] on the one hand, and the federal Drug Abuse Office and Treatment Act of 1972 on the other[19]. •

The conflict between state child abuse reporting laws and state confidentiality laws, by contrast, is only apparent. State legislatures have had the wisdom to resolve the conflict by enacting exceptions as part of the state confidentiality laws. Thus, in Illinois, for example, a statutory exception for 'Disclosure in accordance with Abused and Neglected Child Reporting Act' is part of the Mental Health and Developmental Disabilities Confidentiality Act[30]. Also, a similar express exception is part of the Illinois statutory physician–patient privilege[31].

Some writers suggest that there is no real federal conflict since the federal confidentiality laws do not absolutely prohibit disclosure of drug treatment records and even provide for disclosure avenues, albeit narrow ones, such as patient consent, emergency treatment and appropriate court orders. Upon close scrutiny, none of these exceptions is really that helpful in a setting involving child abuse or neglect resulting from perinatal drug addiction of a mother under treatment. The mother–patient is not likely to give written consent to report child abuse. Consent by the victim–patient in a perinatal setting is inapplicable. The federal regulations governing disclosure for emergency medical treatment do not permit disclosure to child abuse authorities, but only to treating medical personnel. Resorting to court action each time is cumbersome, expensive and has the inherent disincentive of subjecting the mother–patient to involvement in adversarial court proceedings. Anonymous reporting, i.e. not identifying the patient or the fact she is in treatment for addiction, while a technical possibility, is dishonest since inevitably the state authority's investigation will lead to knowledge of the mother–patient's identity and the fact of her treatment for drug addiction.

Happily, the law is evolving quickly toward the predominance of federal and state child abuse and neglect reporting laws over federal confidentiality laws. In contested cases, courts have consistently granted appropriate disclosure orders for the purpose of facilitating the enforcement of child abuse and neglect reporting laws. Such orders have been granted by the New York courts in *In the Matter of the Doe Children*[32], involving a mother enrolled in a methadone program and in *In the Matter of Dwayne G.*[33] where the mother was in an alcoholism counseling program. Also, in *In the Matter of Baby X*[8] involving prenatal and perinatal drug use by the mother, an appropriate disclosure order was granted by the Michigan Appellate Court. In 1984 the Minnesota Supreme Court granted such a disclosure order where the male patient was being treated for alcoholism in *State of Minnesota* v. *David Gerald Andring*[34].

In *Andring*, the Minnesota Supreme Court perceptively pointed out that the conflict was between two federal laws, namely, between the reporting requirements of the Child Abuse Prevention and Treatment Act of 1974[1] and the confidentiality protections under the Comprehensive Alcohol Abuse and Alcoholism Prevention, Treatment, and Rehabilitation Act Amendments of 1974[35]. *Andring* concluded that the federal alcohol treatment Act's and regulations' confidentiality protections do not preempt the state Child Abuse Act[36], and that neither Congress nor the Secretary for the Department of Health and Human Services (HHS), who is charged with administering both federal statutes and their regulations, could have intended that the confidentiality provisions of the alcohol treatment regulations render the child abuse reporting requirements ineffective[37].

Applying the *Andring* court's rationale to the conflict between the confidentiality provisions of the federal Drug Abuse Office and Treatment Act of 1972[19] and the reporting requirements of the federal Child Abuse Prevention and Treatment Act of 1974[1] is readily done.

The US Attorney General's Task Force on Family Violence recommended in 1984 that federal confidentiality statutes and regulations for federal alcohol and drug abuse treatment programs should be amended to require compliance with state laws on mandatory reporting of child abuse, neglect and molestation.

On 18 June 1985, US Senator Alan B. Cranston introduced a bill known as S.1320, observing that the time had come to deal with this conflict problem in a straightforward manner[38]. In part, S.1320 would add the following new subsection (i) to appropriate sections of the Public Health Service Act[39] dealing respectively with confidentiality protections for alcoholism and drug treatment programs:

(i) Nothing in this section shall be construed to supersede the applications of State or local requirements for the reporting of incidents of suspected child abuse to the appropriate State or local authorities.

151

Thus there is a clear trend now in which the interest of protecting child welfare, health and safety through enforcement of the child abuse and neglect reporting laws is predominating over countervailing confidentiality interests. The health care professional should bear that in mind when judging whether to report a suspected case of child abuse or neglect resulting from perinatal addiction.

'BABY DOE' LAWS AND REGULATIONS – MEDICAL NEGLECT

The chief relevance of the 'Baby Doe' laws and regulations to this discussion lies in what they have to say concerning the concept of 'medical neglect' in the care and treatment of newborns, particularly severely defective newborns. The significant incidence of neonatal deficits generated by maternal addiction makes this part of the discussion even more relevant. There are two separate and distinct sets of 'Baby Doe' laws and regulations, each with its respective statutory and regulatory structure. They are referred to hereinafter as 'Baby Doe I' and 'Baby Doe II'.

The statutory basis for Baby Doe I is section 504 of the federal Rehabilitation Act of 1973[40], which provides in pertinent part:

No otherwise qualified handicapped individual in the United States shall, *solely by reason of his handicap,* be excluded from participation in, be denied the benefits of, or be subjected to discrimination under any program or activity receiving Federal assistance. (Emphasis added)

By Presidential Executive Order[41], the Secretary of HHS is directed to establish standards for determining who are handicapped individuals and what are discriminatory practices under section 504 of the Act. The Secretary of HHS did establish such final regulations effective 13 February 1984[42]. In part, these regulations address the responsibilities of state child protective agencies for the reporting to the state and to HHS cases of 'unlawful medical neglect.' HHS was charged with a direct enforcement and investigative role under the Baby Doe I regulations.

The operative principle of the final Baby Doe I regulations is that treatment decisions for handicapped infants be based on reasonable medical judgements, and medically beneficial treatment not be withheld *solely* on the basis of an infant's present or anticipated mental or physical impairments. The federal financial assistance involved, or the jurisdictional bridge, is federal funding of Medicare or state public health care programs such as Medicaid and ICARE in Illinois. The ultimate sanction for a participating provider (physician and/or hospital) would be the loss of provider status under those federally assisted health care programs.

It is interesting to note that as an additional federal statutory basis for the Baby Doe I regulations, HHS asserts the federal Drug Abuse Office and Treatment Act of 1972, discussed above[19]. While the reason for doing so is unclear, the author speculates that HHS sees the connection between addiction and a high incidence of neonatal deficits or handicaps.

152

As of this writing, the Baby Doe I regulations are on appeal before the US Supreme Court. They have been found to be invalid twice by the US Court of Appeals in two separate cases as an unwarranted extension of federal jurisdiction under section 504 of the Rehabilitation Act of 1973[43]. Traditionally, section 504 of the Act has been applied to employment and educational settings. Enforcement of the Baby Doe I regulations is stayed by court order pending the result of the appeal to the US Supreme Court which is expected to sustain their invalidation.

By contrast, the Baby Doe II regulations are in effect. Their federal statutory basis is the Child Abuse Prevention and Treatment Act of 1974 and the Child Abuse Amendments of 1984, again, two of the same laws discussed above[1,2]. The Secretary of HHS established final implementing regulations, the so-called Baby Doe II regulations, effective 9 October 1984[44].

The 1974 Act, as we have seen above, requires the several states to enact and enforce the federal child abuse and neglect reporting and enforcement framework as a condition of continuing to receive federal funding for these programs. The 1984 Amendments, among other things, add a new funding eligibility criterion in the form of a new clause (K) to section 4(b)(2) of the 1974 Act as follows:

Within one year after the date of the enactment of the Child Abuse Amendments of 1984, have in place for the purpose of responding to the reporting of medical neglect (including instances of withholding of medically indicated treatment from disabled infants with life-threatening conditions), procedures or programs, or both (within the State child protective services system), to provide for (i) coordination and consultation with individuals designated by and within appropriate healthcare facilities, (ii) prompt notification by individuals designated by and within appropriate healthcare facilities of cases of suspected medical neglect (including instances of withholding of medically indicated treatment from disabled infants with life-threatening conditions), and (iii) authority, under State law, for the State child protective service system to pursue any legal remedies, including the authority to initiate legal proceedings in a court of competent jurisdiction, as may be necessary to prevent the withholding of medically indicated treatment from disabled infants with life-threatening conditions.

Under the Baby Doe II regulations there is no direct enforcement role for the federal government. The state alone investigates and processes reports of child 'medical neglect', as with any other reported child abuse or neglect.

The following are the highlights of the final Baby Doe II regulations[45]. They define the terms 'medical neglect' and 'withholding of medically indicated treatment' as used in new clause (K) of sections 4(b)(2) and (3) of the 1974 Act. Nutrition, hydration and medication (so-called 'comfort care') are absolute requirements and may not ever be withheld. Other forms of treatment may be withheld based on 'reasonable medical judgment' that *any* of the following exist: (1) the infant is chronically and irreversibly comatose; or (2) treatment would merely prolong the infant's death; or (3) treatment would be virtually futile for the infant's survival and be inhumane.

The sanctions are those provided for individuals convicted of having violated state child abuse laws. For licensed health care professionals, such a final and unappealable conviction can be grounds for licensure sanction up to and including permanent revocation.

NON-VOLUNTARY TREATMENT FOR PERINATAL DRUG ADDICTION – THE EXISTING LEGAL INFRASTRUCTURE

This treatise would be incomplete without suggesting a solution based in law for other than a voluntary treatment mode of perinatal drug addiction because of the high risk of injury to, or death of, the fetus in addition to that of the mother. The basis of the need for such a non-voluntary treatment mode is compellingly articulated in the following excerpt:

> The number of infants born to narcotic-addicted mothers in the United States is estimated at about 9,000 per year and the number of infants exposed to opiates during the perinatal period at 300,000. While early diagnosis and treatment have improved the survival rate of addicted infants, there is evidence to suggest that early exposure of human infants to narcotics is associated with long-lasting somatic and/or psychological deficits in somatic and psychological development. Development has been reported to be within normal range, however, in other studies. A wide range of animal studies has shown sequelae that persist throughout adulthood. Data are also available, primarily from animal studies, which indicate that offspring of males exposed to morphine or methadone may also be at risk, i.e., increased mortality, lower birth weight, learning impairment, and effects that persist into the second generation[46].

A legal infrastructure is already in place upon which such a non-voluntary treatment mode might be based. The elements of this infrastructure are the various aspects of the state's interest and rights in protecting the viable fetus and the neonate. In *Roe* v. *Wade* the US Supreme Court held that the state has an 'important and legitimate interest in protecting the potentiality of human life'[47]. The *Roe* Court then found this interest to predominate over the other competing interests of the mother's right to privacy concerning self-determination over her own body, safeguarding maternal health and maintaining medical standards at the point of fetal viability[48]. The *Roe* Court articulated its determination on this score in the following manner:

> With respect to the State's important and legitimate interest in potential life, the 'compelling' point is viability. This is so because the fetus then

presumably has the capability of meaningful life outside the mother's womb. State regulation protective of fetal life after viability thus has both logical and biological justifications. If the State is interested in protecting fetal life after viability, it may go as far as to proscribe abortion during that period, except when it is necessary to preserve the life or health of the mother[49].

Post-*Roe* US Supreme Court decisions are likewise instructive on this point. In *Mauer* v. *Roe* the Court stated that the 'state unquestionably has a strong and legitimate interest in encouraging normal childbirth' as an interest closely intertwined with its 'direct interest in protecting the fetus'[50]. Likewise, in *Harris* v. *McRae* the Supreme Court held 'that the Hyde Amendment, by encouraging childbirth Bis rationally related to the legitimate governmental objective of protecting potential life'[51].

Additionally the state, under its *parens patriae* powers, can mandate medical care for minors against the parents' wishes. This principle has been followed in both life-saving cases and in non-life-saving, but serious, cases[52].

By 1972 the doctrine of disallowing a child's cause of action for prenatal injury inflicted by third parties was extinct when the Supreme Court of Alabama abandoned that rule in *Huskey* v. *Smith*[53]. Every jurisdiction now permits suits by the subsequently born child against third parties for prenatal injuries.

Approximately one-half of the states have abrogated the parent–child tort immunity doctrine, creating a parental duty of care to avoid injury to the child and a corresponding right of the child to be free of parentally caused injury[54]. Thus, the child's right to be born sound predominates over the parents' right of autonomy where prenatal injury is likely[55].

All of the above considerations support state intervention in requiring an addicted expectant mother to undergo non-voluntary treatment, at least following the point of fetal viability. The high risk of serious injury to, or death of, the fetus as the result of maternal addiction is well documented in the literature and should outweigh considerations of restrictions on the mother's personal liberty. Of course, resort to such intervention by the state should be tempered by the sound judgement of physicians and other health care professionals as to its efficacy in given cases. As one writer has so eloquently put it:

To have power to require birth, but not to protect the soon-to-be-born from injury which will follow it throughout life is inconsistent with the interests of the state and the child in freedom from preventable injury. Allowing intervention protects and fosters both[56].

NOTES AND REFERENCES

1. 42 U. S. C. §5101, *et seq.*
2. P. L. 98 – 457.
3. 45 C. F. R. §1340, *et seq.* Illinois Abused and Neglected Child Reporting Act.
4. Ch. 23, I2051, *et seq.*, Ill. Rev. Stat.

5. The following are key statutory definitions from the Illinois Abused and Neglected Child reporting Act, Ch. 23, I2051, *et seq.*, Ill. Rev. Stat.:

§2053. Definitions.

'Child' means any person under the age of 18 years.

'Department' means Department of Children and Family Services.

'Abused Child' means a child whose parent or immediate family member, or any person responsible for the child's welfare, or any individual residing in the same home as the child, or a parmour of the child's parent:

(a) inflicts, causes to be inflicted, or allows to be inflicted upon such child physical injury, by other than accidental means, which causes death, disfigurement, impairment of physical or emotional health, or loss or impairment of any bodily function;

(b) creates a substantial risk of physical injury to such child by other than accidental means which would be likely to cause death, disfigurement, impairment of physical or emotional health, or loss or impairment of any bodily function;

(c) commits or allows to be committed any sex offense against such child, as such sex offenses are defined in the Criminal Code of 1961, as amended, and extending those definitions of sex offenses to include children under 18 years of age;

(d) commits or allows to be committed an act or acts of torture upon such child; or

(e) inflicts excessive corporal punishment.

'Neglected Child' means any child whose parent *or other person responsible for the child's welfare withholds or denies nourishment or medically indicated treatment including food or care denied solely on the basis of the present or anticipated mental or physical impairment as determined by a physician acting alone or in consultation with other physicians* or otherwise does not provide the proper or necessary support, education as required by law, *or medical or other remedial care* recognized under State law as necessary for a child's well-being, or other care necessary for his or her well-being, including adequate food, clothing and shelter; or who is abandoned by his or her parents or other person responsible for the child's welfare. A child shall not be considered neglected or abused for the sole reason that such child's parent or other person responsible for his or her welfare depends upon spiritual means through prayer alone for the treatment or cure of disease or remedial care as provided under Section 4 of this Act. (Emphasis added)

6. 75 Cal. App. 3d 214, 141 Cal. Rptr. 912 (4th Dist. Ct. 1977).

7. 80 Mich. App. 219, 263 N. W. 2d 37 (1977).

8. 97 Mich. App. 111, 293 N. W. 2d 736 (1980).

9. *Parens patriae* power is the state's limited paternalistic power to protect or promote the welfare of certain individuals like young children who lack the capacity to act in their own best interests. *Development in the Law – The Constitution and the Family,* 93 Harv. L. Rev. 1156, 1199 (1980).

10. *Hoener* v. *Bertinato,* 67 N. J. Supr. 517, 171 A.2d 140 (1961); *Raleigh Fitkin-Paul Morgan Memorial Hospital* v. *Anderson,* 42 N. J. 421, 201 A.2d 537, *cert. denied,* 377 U.S. 985 (1964).

11. *Jefferson* v. *Griffin Spalding County Hospital Authority,* 247 Ga. 86, 274 S. E. 2d 457 (1981).

12. An unreported Colorado juvenile court case. Bowes, W. A. and Selgestad, B. (1981). Fetal versus maternal rights: Medical and legal perspectives. *American Journal of Obstetrics and Gynecology,* **58,** 209 – 14

13. Unreported February, 1982 Cook County, Illinois, Circuit Court case involving Rush-Presbyterian-St. Luke's Hospital of Chicago, Illinois, granting temporary custody of an unborn child for purposes of consent to medical treatment including Caesarean section and blood transfusion. Also, *In the Matter of Mary A. Brownlow,* Case No. 85-M4-680 (1985), Circuit Court of Cook County, Illinois, Fourth Municipal District, ordering blood transfusions for the unborn fetus.

14. Ch. 23, I2054, Ill. Rev. Stat.

15. 1977 Ill. Op. Atty. Gen. No. S-1298.

16. Ch. 111, I4433(22), Ill. Rev. Stat. (Physicians); Ch. 111, I3420(8), Ill. Rev. Stat. (Nurses); Ch. 111, I4922(o), Ill. Rev. Stat. (Podiatrists); Ch. 111, I5316(16), Ill. Rev. Stat. (Psychologists); Ch. 111, I2222(21), Ill. Rev. Stat. (Dentists); Ch. 111, I6315(g), Ill. Rev. Stat. (Social Workers).

17. Ch. 23, I2055, Ill. Rev. Stat.
18. Ch. 23, I2059, Ill. Rev. Stat.
19. 21 U. S. C. §1175, *et seq.*; Sec. 303 of P. L. 93 – 282.
20. 42 C. F. R. Part 2, §§21 – 2.67 – 1.
21. 21 U. S. C. §1175(a).
22. 21 U. S. C. §1175(b)(1).
23. 21 U. S. C. §1175(b)(2)(A).
24. 21 U. S. C. §1175(b)(2)(B).
25. 21 U. S. C. §1175(b)(2)(C).
26. 21 U. S. C. §1175(f).
27. Roach, W. H., Jr., Chernoff, S. N. and Esley, C. L. (1985). *Medical Records and the Law*, pp. 30 – 35, 72 – 76. (An Aspen Publication)
28. Ch. 91½, I801 *et seq.*, Ill. Rev. Stat.
29. Ch. 110, I8 – 802, Ill. Rev. Stat.
30. Ch. 91½, I811 (i), Ill. Rev. Stat.
31. Ch. 110, I8 – 802, exception (7), Ill. Rev. Stat.
32. 402 N. Y. S. 2d 958 (1978).
33. 411 N. Y. S. 2d 180 (1978).
34. 342 N. W. 2d 128 (1984).
35. 42 U. S. C. §4582.
36. 342 N. W. 2d 128, 131 (1984).
37. 342 N. W. 2d 128, 132 (1984).
38. Fed. Reg. for June 18, 1985 – Vol. 131, No. 81.
39. 42 U. S. C. §290 dd–3 (alcohol treatment); 42 U. S. C. §290 ee–3 (drug treatment).
40. 29 U. S. C. §794.
41. Executive Order 11914.
42. 45 C. F. R. §84.
43. *U. S.* v. *University Hospital, et al.*, 729 F.2d 144; *American Hospital Association, et al.*, v. *Margaret M. Heckler, et al.*, Case No. CA 83 – 774 (USCA−2, 1983); *cert.* granted 105 Supr. Ct. 3475 (1984), Docket Nos. 84 – 1529, 84 – 6211, 84 – 6213.
44. 45 C. F. R. §1340.
45. 45 C. F. R. §1340.15.
46. Morris, R. A. and Sonderegger, T. B. (1984). Legal applications and implications for neurotoxin research of the developing organism. *Neurobehavioral Toxicology and Teratology,* **6,** 303 – 306
47. 410 U. S. 113, 162, (1973).
48. 410 U. S. at 163 – 64.
49. Ibid.
50. 432 U. S. 464, 478 (1977).
51. 478 U. S. 297, 301 and 325 (1980).
52. *In Re Sampson,* 317 N. Y. S. 2d 641, 278 N. E.2d 918 (1972); *People ex rel. Wallace* v. *Labrenz,* 411, Ill. 618, 104 N. E. 2d 769 (Ill. Supr. Ct. 1952); *Wisconsin* v. *Yoder,* 406 U. S. 205 (1972); See also, notes 9, 10 and 11.
53. 289 Ala. 52, 54, 265 So.2d 596, 596 (1972).
54. Simon, C. A. (1978). Parental liability for prenatal injury. *Columbia Journal of Law and Social Problems,* **14,** 47 – 92
55. *Prince* v. *Massachusetts,* 321 U. S. 158 (1944); Levine, M. (1974). The right of the fetus to be born free of drug addiction. *U. C. D. Law Journal,* **7,** 45 – 55
56. Myers, J. E. B. (1984). Abuse and neglect of the unborn: Can the state intervene? *Duq. Law Rev.,* **23,** No. 1, 1 – 76

Index